Neuroimaging of Covid-19. First Insights based on Clinical Cases

Simonetta Gerevini
Editor

Neuroimaging of Covid-19. First Insights based on Clinical Cases

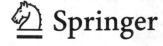 Springer

Editor
Simonetta Gerevini
Neuroradiology Department
Papa Giovanni XXIII Hospital
Bergamo
Italy

ISBN 978-3-030-67523-3   ISBN 978-3-030-67521-9   (eBook)
https://doi.org/10.1007/978-3-030-67521-9

This Springer imprint is published by the registered company Springer Nature Switzerland AG
The registered company address is: Gewerbestrasse 11, 6330 Cham, Switzerland

Acknowledgements

We would like to thank the neuroradiology department of Papa Giovanni XXIII hospital: medical doctors, technicians, nurses and all the professional figures for their work and abnegation as usual, but specifically in this pandemic period. We also wish to thank Cristina Casalini and Antonio Castaldello for their support in acquiring, selecting and preparing the images. Without their assistance, this book would not have been possible.

Contents

1 Introduction... 1
Simonetta Gerevini

2 Background.. 3
Maria Sessa, Marco Rizzi, and Simonetta Gerevini

3 Vascular Manifestations in COVID 19..................... 17
Antonino Barletta, Maria Luisa Colleoni, Luca Quilici,
Gabriele Gallizioli, and Simonetta Gerevini

**4 Posterior Reversible Encephalopathy Syndrome (PRES)
and Meningo-Encephalitis in COVID**..................... 39
Ornella Manara, Giulio Pezzetti, and Simonetta Gerevini

**5 Possible Thrombotic Microangiopathy Occurring in Patient
with CNS Localization of SARS-Cov-2**.................... 69
Simonetta Gerevini, Angela Napolitano, Mariangela Cava,
Emilio Giazzi, and Cristina Agostinis

**6 Still to Be Explored: Involvement of Other
Districts/Organs in COVID-19 Patients**................... 81
Simonetta Gerevini

7 Brain Imaging Findings in COVID-19 Positive Newborns..... 83
Ornella Manara, Antonino Barletta, Giulio Pezzetti,
and Simonetta Gerevini

8 Cardiac Involvement in COVID-19 Infection............... 87
Giulio Guagliumi, Dario Pellegrini, Aloke Finn,
and Simonetta Gerevini

**9 The Neuropathology Spectrum in Deceased Patients
with COVID-19**.. 91
Eleonora Aronica and Simonetta Gerevini

Introduction

Simonetta Gerevini

In December 2019, an outbreak caused by a novel coronavirus (2019-nCoV), now named severe acute respiratory syndrome coronavirus 2 (SARS-CoV-2), occurred in China and has rapidly spread all over the world causing a pandemic. The disease caused by SARS-CoV-2 was named COVID-19. In Europe, the first case was reported in the Lombardy region. Although soon after all Italian regions reported patients with COVID-19, the highest number of cases was in Eastern Lombardy, specifically in the area of Bergamo with 11,313 confirmed COVID-19 patients up to April 30th 2020. For this reason, we decide to explore the known CNS manifestation of this virus, showing the "typical" MRI aspect. In this Atlas we will show real cases we faced in the first outbreak between March and May 2020. COVID-19 may affect CNS presenting with several patterns, nowadays we are trying to define what is typical and what it is not. Therefore, we have separated chapters according to different types of presentation (vascular lesions, inflammatory lesions and so on) and for this reason some topics will be treated extensively in the first chapter and more shortly in each specific other chapter.

1.1 How to Read the Atlas

On the introduction of each chapter you will find some general information on each topic, followed by clinical picture and images sorted to show the lesions in different shapes, sizes, and locations. It should be noted that our intent was not to elaborate on all the details on each case. There may be several different findings but we have tried to demonstrate the most important ones according to the topic. When possible and disposable the entire clinical history of the patient was given in the legend, if not possible due to the fast progression of the disease in that phase of the pandemic, only the specific neurological presentation according to imaging findings were given. We present cases as we faced them in the acute phase of the pandemic.

S. Gerevini (✉)
Neuroradiology Department, Papa Giovanni XXIII Hospital, Bergamo, Italy
e-mail: sgerevini@asst-pg23.it

Maria Sessa, Marco Rizzi, and Simonetta Gerevini

Human coronaviruses, first characterized in the 1960s, are responsible for a substantial proportion of upper respiratory tract infections in children, with occasional cases of pneumonia in infants and young adults; for a few decades since their first identification, their pathogenicity has been considered to be low; non-respiratory localizations of the disease, including neurological complications, have been described as uncommon events [1]. In the new millennium, new more virulent coronaviruses made their appearance in humans SARS-CoV, causing the Severe Acute Respiratory Syndrome (2002–2004) and MERS-CoV, causing the Middle Eastern Respiratory Syndrome (2012–ongoing); also SARS-CoV and MERS-CoV were mostly associated to respiratory disease, but different organs and body systems could be involved, including the Central Nervous System [2], as recently summarized by Verstrepen et al. [3].

The newest human coronavirus, SARS-CoV-2, shares with the other coronaviruses the respiratory route of entry, and the involvement of the respiratory system is the most striking clinical feature; still, there is clear evidence that the disease caused by SARS-CoV-2 (COVID-19, Corona Virus Disease 2019) is a systemic disease, which may involve many different organs and systems.

The clinical spectrum of COVID-19 is very wide, ranging from asymptomatic infection to severe pneumonia with respiratory failure, multi-organ damage and death. While many aspects of the pathogenesis of COVID-19 remain unclarified, it seems to be widely accepted that the most severe cases of the disease may be the result of a multistep pathogenetic process, with a first phase of viral invasion and replication, which in a few cases may progress towards a stage characterized by hyperinflammation (the "cytokine storm") and hypercoagulability (and the consequent thrombotic and thromboembolic events) [4, 5].

M. Sessa
Neurology Unit, Papa Giovanni XXIII Hospital, Bergamo, Italy
e-mail: msessa@asst-pg23.it

M. Rizzi
Infectious Diseases Unit, Papa Giovanni XXIII Hospital, Bergamo, Italy
e-mail: mrizzi@asst-pg23.it

S. Gerevini (✉)
Neuroradiology Department, Papa Giovanni XXIII Hospital, Bergamo, Italy
e-mail: sgerevini@asst-pg23.it

2.1 Pathogenesis of COVID-19 Infection

ACE2 has been identified as the main host cell receptor for SARS-CoV-2; it has been demonstrated that the virus binds to the Angiotensin Converting Enzyme 2 (ACE2) receptor via its spike protein; following binding, processing by transmembrane protease serine 2 (TMPRSS2) and furin conduce to viral entry [6, 7]; the down-regulation of ACE2 that follows viral binding and entry increases the levels of angiotensin II, with its proinflammatory effects (macrophage activation, increased production and release of IL-6, TNF and other cytokines). On the other hand, ACE2 is mostly expressed by alveolar type II cells, which produce the surfactant, and are the progenitors for AT1 cells (the major constituents of the alveolar cellular lining); SARS-CoV-2, binding to ACE2 and entering AT2 cells, kills AT2 cells, induce a surfactant deficit, and injures the alveolar epithelium. The combined effect of inflammatory activation and alveolar damage may result in a state of hyperinflammation which in a few patients may lead to progressive lung damage and full blown Acute Respiratory Distress Syndrome (ARDS), independently of the persistence of viral replication [8].

During the SARS epidemic (2002–2004) it was demonstrated that SARS-CoV bound to ACE2 receptor [6]. And a number of studies were conducted on the distribution of ACE2 receptors in the human body: it has been shown that ACE2 mRNA is present in almost all organs, but its protein expression is mostly present in lung alveolar cells, enterocytes of the small intestine, arterial and venous endothelial cells and arterial smooth muscle cells: this distribution of ACE2 may be of relevance with regard to the multiorgan manifestations of COVID-19 [9].

More recent studies on SARS-CoV-2 have demonstrated a high density of ACE2 in the oral and anal mucosae, the heart and the kidney [10].

Postmortem studies have demonstrated the presence of significant amount of SARS-CoV-2 in lungs, kidneys, liver, heart, bone marrow and brain [11–15].

2.1.1   Hyperinflammation

As previously mentioned, following the initial phase of viral replication, a few patients develop an inflammatory response, which in a few most severe cases may be strikingly intense (the so-called cytokine storm) and may lead to vascular hyperpermeability, organ failure and death. Among the immunological features which have been associated with unfavorable outcomes are increased cytokine levels (IL-6, IL-10, and TNF-α), lymphopenia (in CD4+ and CD8+ T cells), and decreased IFN-γ expression in CD4+ T cells [16–18]. On the basis of this evidence, therapeutic strategies have been developed targeting the immune activation: this has included anti-cytokine therapies (such as tocilizumab and sarilumab, targeting the IL-6 receptor, siltuximab, targeting IL-6, anakinra, targeting the IL-1 receptor, eculizumab, an anti-complement agent,) and immunomodulators (such as steroids or colchicine) have been tested, with conflicting results. As of September 30, 2020, conclusive positive results were only available for the use of dexamethasone [19].

2.1.2   Hypercoagulability

The pathogenesis of hypercoagulability in COVID-19 is still ill-defined. Some experts have postulated that endothelial injury plays a central role in the pathogenesis of acute respiratory distress syndrome and organ failure in patients with severe COVID-19 [20, 21].

There is evidence of direct invasion of endothelial cells by SARS-CoV-2, potentially leading to cell injury [22, 23].

On the other end, endothelial injury may be mediated by cytokines, such as interleukin 4 (IL-4), interleukin 6 (IL-6), interleukin 10 (IL-10), Tumor Necrosis Factor (TNF-1), and other acute phase reactants. The contribution of complement-mediated endothelial injury has also been suggested [24] and experimental COVID-19 therapies targeting these pathogenetic mechanisms have been proposed; there is some preliminary evidence in favor of the use of narsoplimab, a human monoclonal antibody targeting mannan-binding lectin-associated serine protease-2. Narsoplimab, which is approved for the treatment of Hematopoietic Stem Cell Transplant-associated Thrombotic MicroAngiopathy (HSCT-TMA) and atypical Hemolytic Uremic Syndrome (aHUS) down-modulates SARS-CoV-2-induced activation of the lectin pathway and endothelial cell damage, and could reduce the thrombotic risk of COVID-19 patients [25].

Despite a growing evidence that prothrombotic factors may present high circulating levels in patients with severe COVID-19: this has been observed for D-dimer, fibrinogen, von Willebrand factor, factor VIII, and the well-known frequency and severity of thrombotic events in COVID-19, the best therapeutical approach to anticoagulation remain ill-defined.

2.1.3 A Few Final Remarks on the Pathogenesis of COVID-19

While a large amount of data have been collected on hyperinflammation and the "cytokine storm" in the COVID-19 literature, many points remain to be clarified; recently it has been noted that when cytokines levels are measured in COVID-19, they may not result as high as observed in other common conditions, such as sepsis/septic shock, burns and non-COVID-19 related ARDS [26, 27]. This obviously would have great implications for the treatment protocols who aim at downregulating the host inflammatory response in order to prevent organ damage and disease progression: in fact, so far anti-inflammatory treatments have proven of dubious or limited efficacy. In general, the objective of a reduction of the immune response is a tricky one: a well-balanced inflammatory response and coagulation activation are to some degree necessary for pathogen clearance. It should be noted that while a number of biological markers have been investigated as potential tools for the monitoring of inflammation and of the activation of the coagulation pathways (from C-Reactive-Protein to Interleukin 6 to D-dimer), there is still a lack of consensus on the use of these markers in clinical care.

It seems reasonable to argue that we need to greatly improve our ability to identify the different phases of the disease (viral invasion and replication, immune response and hyperinflammation, hypercoagulability and thrombotic events), the degree of immune activation, and the different level of organs involvement, so as to be able to make use of finely tuned treatment protocols.

Finally, with regard to the pathogenesis of COVID-19, it has to be noted that the disease is not "switched off" at discharge or whenever the acute phase symptoms subside: the issue of "long-hauling COVID-19" is very much debated; the first available data from follow up studies show that a number of patients still have symptoms a few months after the acute phase, and in some of these patients there is laboratory evidence of persisting immune activation and hypercoagulability; in a series of 743 patients from the Bergamo hospital, at a median of 105 days from symptoms onset, 290 persons (39%) still had raised D-dimer values. This may signal an active disease, with a risk for disease progression and organ damage, including acute severe events, such as major thrombotic episodes; may be that some patients may well deserve some kind of mid-long-term treatment (anti-inflammatory, anticoagulant) in order to reduce the risk of unfavorable outcomes. Much more research is needed in this field.

2.2 Neurological Manifestations in SARS-CoV-2 Infection

Growing evidence indicates that the novel coronavirus disease 2019 (COVID-19) is not limited to the respiratory system and that SARS-CoV-2 has an organotropism beyond the respiratory tract, including the brain. After the first cases of COVID-19 were reported in Wuhan, China, in December 2019, an increasing numbers of case reports and case series report neurological and neuropsychiatric syndromes associated with the disease. However, much is still unknown about their frequency, accurate characteristics, pathophysiology, risk factors, and prognosis.

2.2.1 Neurological Manifestations in Other Types of Coronavirus

Up to date, several reports have described the association between respiratory viral infections sustained by different human respiratory virus [syncytial virus (hRSV), the influenza virus (IV), the human metapneumovirus (hMPV), as well as the coronavirus (CoV)] with neurological symptoms.

Involvement of both Peripheral Nervous System (PNS) and Central Nervous System CNS has been reported in patients with SARS- and MERS-CoV infections, mostly developing 2–4 weeks after onset of respiratory symptoms.

Neuromuscular involvement has been described in three patients with SARS, including polyneuropathy, myopathy and rhabdomyolysis [28–30].

Additional cases of peripheral and overlap syndromes have been described in MERS including critical illness neuropathy, Guillain-Barré Syndrome, Bickerstaff's brainstem encephalitis, and toxins (including drugs) or virus-related sensory neuropathy [31, 32].

Ischemic stroke has been described both in SARS [33] and in MERS [34], as well as hemorrhagic stroke in MERS [31].

Altered level of consciousness ranging from confusion to coma, associated with MERS-CoV had been described in three patients. Brain magnetic resonance revealed striking changes characterized by widespread, bilateral hyperintense lesions on T2-weighted imaging within the white matter and subcortical areas without gadolinium enhancement, whose characteristics were suggestive of acute disseminated leukoencephalopathy, acute infarction, and encephalitis, respectively [34].

2.2.2 Neurological Manifestation: Experience with Novel SARS-CoV-2 Infection

2.2.2.1 Epidemiology

Prevalence of neurological manifestations in SARS-CoV-2 infection is highly variable ranging from 3.5% up to 84%. However, the precise evaluation of incidence and prevalence is undermined by a series of methodological issues.

First of all, "neurological symptoms" are not precisely categorized. In some reports nonspecific complaints based on subjective descriptions,

such as dizziness, have been included [35, 36]. In the subsequent publications, nonspecific symptoms likely due to the systemic condition and neurologic symptom fully accounted for by sedation were either excluded or properly classified.

Except for Karadas study all studies were retrospective and data regarding neurologic complications derived from medical records; either mild symptoms or neurological manifestations in highly compromised patients may have been underestimated.

Data were collected either from limited or selected cohort. Helms reports the neurological features of patients with severe ARDS admitted in intensive care units (ICUs) [37]; Paterson's cases were discussed in the context of multidisciplinary team meeting, thus representing a bias toward more complex and severe cases [38]; Benussi reports clinical characteristics of patients admitted to a neuro-COVID Unit with neurological disease, excluding therefore all neurological complications occurring in COVID patients hospitalized in other wards and ICUs [39] in the only nation-based study [40], voluntary-based case notification might have been under-reported because of the clinical demands of the pandemic.

Instrumental evaluations were not systematically performed either to reduce the risk of cross infection [35] or likely due to the well-known difficulties in transferring patients admitted in ICU for instrumental tests [37].

In the three studies analyzing the main neurological diagnosis/syndromes conducted on all patients with confirmed COVID-19 disease admitted to tertiary care designated COVID-19 hospitals [41–43] the prevalence was 7.7%, 3.5%, and 7.8% respectively.

Finally, as these studies were hospital based, they do not necessarily reflect the true incidence of neurological manifestations in individuals with SARS-CoV-2 infection in the community. The stay-at-home recommendations/orders and the general fear for the hospital during the COVID-19 pandemic may have prevented patients from presenting to the hospital, in particular older patients and patients with small deficits and mild symptoms.

2.2.2.2 Neuro-Invasiveness and Neurotropism of SARS-CoV-2

An open question remains if the neurological manifestations reported in patients with SARS-CoV-2 infection represent coincidental occurrence, common complications during severe infectious disease, or a direct consequence of the viral infection. In the latter case, nervous system damage may either be a consequence of direct viral penetration or secondary to indirect para-infective mechanisms.

Several routes of CNS invasion can be used by viral pathogens, among which the hematogenous route or the neurological route through peripheral nerves or olfactory sensory neurons [44].

Similar to SARS-CoV, COVID-19 virus exploits the angiotensin converting enzyme 2 (ACE2) receptor to gain entry inside the cells. ACE2 receptors are widely distributed on the surface of different cells, among which endothelial cells, neurons, and glial cells. Once in the general circulation SARS-CoV-2 pass into the cerebral circulation and interacts with ACE2 receptors expressed in the capillary endothelium. Subsequent damage of the endothelial lining may be responsible of the viral access to the brain and interaction with ACE2 receptors expressed on neurons and glial cells [45].

Neuro-invasiveness possibly via the olfactory nerves had been already demonstrated for other coronavirus. Experimental studies using transgenic mice revealed that either SARS-CoV [46] or MERS-COV [47] when given intranasally could enter the brain, possibly via the olfactory nerves, and thereafter rapidly spread to some specific brain areas including thalamus and brainstem. In mice inoculated intranasally with avian influenza virus [48], viral antigens have been detected in the nucleus of the solitary tract and nucleus ambiguus of the brainstem, The nucleus of the solitary tract receives sensory information from the mechanoreceptors and chemoreceptors in the lung and respiratory tracts [49]; efferent fibers from the nucleus ambiguus and the nucleus of the solitary tract provide innervation to airway smooth muscle, glands, and blood vessels. These interconnections may provide the neuroanatomic basis of cardiorespiratory dysfunction in COVID-19 patients.

Direct demonstration of viral colonization of CNS in patients infected by coronavirus is scarce. HCoV OC43 has been found in the brain tissue sample obtained from a child with fatal encephalitis [50]. The first demonstration of the entry of SARS-CoV into the CNS was obtained through real-time reverse transcription Polymerase Chain Reaction (RT-PCR) assay targeting the polymerase region (orf1ab polyprotein) of the SARS-CoV genome in the CSF of a SARS patient with status epilepticus [51]. Autoptic studies on the samples from patients with SARS have demonstrated the presence of SARS-CoV particles in the brain [52, 53]. In two out of the three patients described by Arabi with altered level of consciousness, in whom CSF analysis was performed, MERS-CoV RT-PCR was negative [34].

The detection of SARS-CoV-2 RNA in the CSF by RT-PCR in COVID-19 patients is quite rare. Since the first report in a patient with meningoencephalitis [54], only few additional cases have been described [55–57].

Conclusive pathological demonstrations of the presence of SARS-CoV-2 in the CNS are missing. At postmortem examinations of ten COVID-19 patients, no signs of encephalitis or central nervous system vasculitis were found and RT-PCR for SARS-CoV-2 was negative in all CSF samples [58].

From an autopsy series of 27 patients quantification of the SARS-CoV-2 viral load by RT-PCR in multiple organs detected SARS-CoV-2 copies at low level per cell also in the brain [13].

Sampling was obtained from brains of 18 patients who died 0–32 days after the onset of symptoms of COVID-19, all of whom, according to a retrospective chart review by neurologists, presented a state of confusion or decreased arousal from sedation for ventilation. Brain magnetic resonance imaging, electroencephalogram, and cerebrospinal fluid examinations were not performed. Histopathological examination showed only hypoxic changes and did not show encephalitis or other specific brain changes referable to the virus. There was no cytoplasmic viral staining on immunohistochemical analysis. The virus was detected at low levels in six brain sections obtained from five patients [59].

Electron microscopy studies showed intracytoplasmic vacuoles containing virus-like particles in neural and capillary endothelial cells from frontal lobe brain sections [60] and a spherical particle with size suspicious for a viral particle in the medulla oblongata.

2.2.2.3 Neurological Manifestations

Cerebrovascular Disease (CVD)

Numerous pathogenic mechanisms contributing to COVID-19 related cerebrovascular syndromes have been proposed. Consistent haemostatic changes in COVID-19 patients, primarily thrombocytopenia and elevated D-dimer levels, indicate some forms of coagulopathy that may predispose to thrombotic events. Nevertheless, it is yet unknown whether these haemostatic changes are a specific effect of SARS-CoV-2 or are a consequence of the cytokine storm [61]. Besides the more common haemostatic alterations, the presence of antiphospholipid antibodies has been reported in some small case series [62–64].

In addition, severe endothelial injury associated with intracellular SARS-CoV-2 virus and disrupted endothelial cell membranes as well as widespread vascular thrombosis with microangiopathy and occlusion of alveolar capillaries have been described in the lungs [65] and might also occur in the brain. Finally, SARS-CoV-2 might be responsible of a true vasculitic process.

CVD, in particular acute ischemic stroke (AIS), is emerging as a frequent complication of SARS-CoV-2 infection. Across five studies with a total of 4466 COVID-19 pts [35, 37, 66–68]. AIS was reported in 54 pts, yielding an overall pooled incidence of 1.2%. Studies were conducted in different countries (France, Netherlands, Italy, China, and the United States) with varying ethnic demographics. Two studies had patient cohorts specifically consisting of patients with severe COVID-19 infection, three included all hospitalized patients with laboratory proven COVID-19 infection [69]. In the Bergamo cohort, CVD represented 38.7% of all neurological

manifestations, 70% of which were AIS [43]. The reported median age ranged from 63.4 [69] to 71.2 years [70]. At binary logistic regression analysis comparing AIS COVID positive patients with COVID negative contemporary controls and historical controls, age did not resulted significantly associated with COVID status [68]. Available literature suggests that stroke in COVID positive patients have a higher severity estimated by the National Institute of Health Stroke Scale (NIHSS). In the systematic review and meta-summary of Tan [69] mean NIHHS value was 19. Yagi reported a median value of 19 significantly associated with COVID status at binary logistic regression analysis comparing AIS COVID positive patients with COVID negative contemporary controls and historical controls. In the Global COVID Stroke Registry the median NIHSS was 10 (IQR: 4–18), and in the 1:1 matched sample of 336 patients with and without COVID-19, the NIHSS was higher in patients with COVID-19 [70]. High NIHSS values are consistent with the frequent observation of large vessel occlusion in a sistematic review [69], large cohort [68], registry [70] and in case series [63].

Available data suggest a poor overall outcome either in terms of in-hospital mortality or residual severe functional deficits assessed by mean of modified Rankin Scale (mRS). Mortality ranged from to 28% in the Global COVID-19 Stroke Registry to 63% in the stroke population admitted to three comprehensive stroke centers in New York. Among 96 survivors with available information about disability status, 49 (51%) had severe disability at discharge. In the propensity score matched population ($n = 330$), patients with COVID-19 had higher risk for severe disability (median mRS 4 [IQR: 2–6] versus 2 [IQR: 1–4], $p < 0.001$) and death (odds ratio, 4.3 [95% CI, 2.22–8.30]) compared with patients with non-COVID-19. Similarly, in the Brescia cohort, patients with COVID-19 had higher mRS scores at discharge with a significantly lower number of patients with a good outcome [39].

Besides stroke-related factors, such as large vessel occlusion, other several potential explanations can account for the increased stroke severity and poor outcome, among which the multi-system complications of COVID-19, including acute cardiac injury and cardiac arrhythmias, acute respiratory distress syndrome, pulmonary embolism, shock, cytokine release syndrome, secondary infection [71].

In addition, the prolonged mechanical ventilation and intensive care unit stay renders patients vulnerable to complications such as hypotension and inadequate cerebral perfusion, superimposed bacterial infection with septic embolization, stress cardiomyopathy, and atrial fibrillation, which represent independent factors for poor prognosis.

Limited data are available concerning outcomes after reperfusion therapies. In the Global COVID-19 Stroke Registry 12 out of 21 (57%) patients treated with intravenous recombinant tissue plasminogen activator (rt-PA) had poor outcome compared to 45% in the non-COVID-19 population registered in the Acute Stroke Registry and Analysis of Lausanne (ASTRAL Registry) between 2003 and 2019. From the same Global COVID-19 Stroke Registry, 11/12 and 8/8 patients treated with thrombolysis plus thrombectomy or with primary endovascular thrombectomy respectively had poor outcome, compared to 3/12 and 3/6 in the ASTRAL Registry [70]. Benussi reported a significant lower number of patients with good outcome in the COVID-19 group, difference that was also confirmed considering only patients who underwent acute phase therapies. Similarly, overall poor outcome is reported in small case series of patients undergoing mechanical thrombectomy [72, 73].

On the opposite, Rifino reported the case of a 66-year-old woman with basilar artery thrombosis treated with intravenous alteplase followed by a first mechanical thrombectomy with excellent angiographic and clinical outcome, and a second successful thrombectomy, the following day, for the acute occlusion of the M1 segment of right middle cerebral artery.

The STROKOVID network, a joint initiative of ten stroke hub centers in Lombardy region, is collecting comprehensive information on patients hospitalized for acute ischemic stroke in Lombardy during SARS-CoV-2 outbreak and is expected to address clinical and research questions.

Even if less frequent, intracranial hemorrhages have been reported [36, 39, 41]. Out of 755 COVID-19 positive adult patients with available neuroimaging, radiographic evidence of ICH was present in 33. It is of note that, based on review by the study neuroradiologist, 26/33 bleeds were considered to have suffered hemorrhagic conversion of an ischemic infarct [74].

Single cases of cerebral venous thrombosis have been described, especially in young patients [75–77].

Encephalopathies, Disorders of Consciousness, Altered Mental Status

Patients presenting with impaired vigilance, confusion and disorientation, psychosis, seizures are commonly described [36, 37, 40, 41, 43] with a very different prevalence values ranging from 9.6% up to 65%. The exact prevalence of these manifestations is limited by the above-mentioned methodological issues, mainly represented by the different cohorts evaluated, and the limited access to diagnostic, which makes very likely that different nosological entities are included in this category.

In the ALBACOVID Registry disorders of consciousness were the most observed neurologic symptoms (19.6%), especially in the severe COVID-19 group and in the advanced stages of COVID-19 disease. These manifestations were statistically associated with older age [78]. In Paterson's series patients were mostly >50 years, neuroimaging was within normal limits, and CSF studies were normal when performed [38].

Inflammatory CNS Syndromes

By definition, encephalitis is an inflammatory process with diagnostic supportive evidences, which include the presence of a CSF pleocytosis and elevated protein, MRI consistent with inflammation, seizures on electroencephalogram. However, in the majority of the CSF samples obtained from COVID-19 patients with clinical presentation suggestive of encephalitis, signs of inflammation are modest or even absent [37, 38,

78]. Experimental data on transgenic mice expressing the human SARS-CoV receptor, where viral entry in CNS was associated with neuronal injury, but relatively limited inflammation, support real-life observations [46].

Definitive evidence of viral neuro-invasion would include a positive CSF RT-PCR for SARS-CoV-2, intrathecal synthesis of SARS-CoV-2-specific antibodies, or detection of SARS-CoV-2 antigen or RNA in brain tissue.

Encephalitis Resulting from Direct SARS-CoV-2 Spreading to the CNS

Cases meeting strict criteria for encephalitis resulting from direct SARS-CoV-2 spreading to the CNS are currently two [54, 79, 80].

Para-Infective and Post-infective Encephalitis in the Absence of CNS Viral Invasion

More frequent are the description of cases with inflammatory features in the absence of CNS viral invasion, which raises the possibility that some cases of COVID-19 inflammatory encephalopathies could result from immune-mediated mechanisms.

Two patients were described with nuchal rigidity, altered mental status, mild CSF lymphocytic pleocytosis (17–21 cells/μL^3) and elevated CSF protein (46–47 mg/dL), negative RCSF T-PCR for SARS-CoV-2, and normal MRI [81].

Pilotto et al. describe a 60-year-old man with confusion, irritability, apathy progressing to "akinetic mutism" and nuchal rigidity, with improvement coincident to administration of high dose methylprednisolone. The CSF showed a mild lymphocytic pleocytosis (18 cells/μL^3), elevated protein (70 mg/dL), and RT-PCR negative twice for SARS-CoV-2. An EEG showed generalized slowing. The CT and MRI were normal [82].

Six patients with severe ARDS and depressed consciousness and/or agitation were considered to have "autoimmune meningoencephalitis". CSF cellularity was normal in all patients and protein level was elevated in five (52–131 mg/dL). In three patients MRI showed cortical hyperintensities with sulcal effacement. Patients were felt to have responded to plasma exchange [83].

Paterson described one patient with opsoclonus, stimulus sensitive myoclonus and convergence spasm, in whom a diagnosis of autoimmune brainstem encephalitis, despite brain imaging, EEG and CSF were normal, and a second patient with confusion and a single seizure, with MRI abnormalities suggestive of autoimmune or 'limbic' encephalitis in the thalami, medial temporal regions and pons [38].

Seven cases of encephalitis no further characterized are described in a UK-surveillance study on neurological and neuropsychiatric complications of COVID-19 [40].

In Paterson's series nine patients were categorized within the spectrum of ADEM. Four patients had hemorrhagic change on imaging and one had necrosis; two patients had myelitis in addition to brain imaging changes. Brain biopsy from one patient, performed at the time of decompressive craniectomy showed evidence of perivenular inflammation supporting aggressive hyper-acute ADEM. A full clinical response was seen in 1 of 12, partial recovery at the time of writing in 10 of 12, and one patient died. Treatments were with corticosteroids in nine, and IVIG in three. Despite the severe imaging findings, the CSF parameters were abnormal in only half. When tested, specific antibodies to NMDAR, MOG, AQP4, LGI1, or GAD were absent in the serum or CSF.

Additional Cases of Acute Demyelinating Encephalomyelitis (ADEM) and Acute Necrotizing Encephalitis (ANE) have been reported. Whenever tested, CSF studies were unremarkable including negative RT-PCR for SARS-CoV-2 [84, 85].

Twenty-five cases of encephalitis in COVID-19 patients were included in the ENCOVID multicenter study recruited from 13 centers in northern Italy. CSF showed hyper proteinorrachia and/or pleocytosis in 68% of cases whereas SARS-CoV-2 RNA by RT-PCR resulted negative. Based on MRI, cases were classified as ADEM, limbic encephalitis, encephalitis with normal imaging and encephalitis with MRI alterations. ADEM and limbic encephalitis cases showed a delayed onset compared to the other encephalitis and were associated with previous more severe COVID-19 respiratory involvement. Patients with MRI alterations exhibited worse response to treatment and final outcomes compared to other encephalitis [86].

An increasing number of acute myelitis is accumulating. In all of them, when tested, RT-PCR for SARS-CoV-2 in cerebrospinal fluid (CSF) was negative. Except for the case of one patient, dead for cardiac arrest [87] in all other cases a good response to iv steroid has been reported [88–90].

A case of acute necrotizing myelitis has been also described [91].

An additional case presenting with acute flaccid paralysis of bilateral lower limbs and sphincter incontinence has been described. However, no CSF analysis nor spinal magnetic resonance images (MRI) were performed, making diagnosis of myelitis presumptive [92].

Rifino reports two cases of myelitis, in whom extensive work-up excluded known causes of myelitis RT-PCR for SARS-CoV2 in CSF was negative. However, CSF IgG antibodies to SARS-CoV2 were present in both patients. Due to their clinical history of fever, the evidence of blood IgG anti-SARS-CoV2, and the lag-time between the onset of COVID-19 symptoms and neurological manifestations, a post-infectious aetiology has been proposed. In only one previous case IgG antibodies to SARS-CoV2 were tested in CSF, and no specific intrathecal synthesis of Anti-SARS-CoV IgG was present [90].

In two cases, myelitis was associated with acute motor axonal neuropathy (AMAN). In one report, the patient was treated with methylprednisolone 1 g IV for 5 days without improvements. Signs of peripheral neuropathy appeared 3 weeks after her initial onset of symptoms. Spinal fluid analysis and EMG confirmed the diagnosis of AMAN. The patient received five rounds of plasma exchange and started to make some clinical recovery 4–5 weeks after her clinical presentation [93]. In a second case, AMAN was associated with myelitis and anti-GD1b positivity after SARS-CoV-2 infection. The patient underwent plasma exchange followed by one course of intravenous immunoglobulins, partially recovering the strength in the upper limbs [94].

Finally, one case of Myelin Oligodendrocyte Glycoprotein Antibody–Associated Optic Neuritis and Myelitis has been described with excellent recover after iv steroid [95].

Peripheral Neurological Disorders

Loss of smell and taste is the most frequently reported symptoms resulting from involvement of the PNS in patients with COVID-19. A recent meta-analysis has shown that anosmia/hyposmia/dysomia and ageusia/hypogcusia/dysgeusia have an estimated global prevalence of 48% and 41% in patients with COVID-19, respectively. Both symptoms may affect one third of patients. These can manifest in the early stages of viral infection, even in pauci symptomatic patients and can persist over time, after the acute phase of the disease [96].

After the first reports of Guillain-Barré syndrome [97–99] numerous additional case reports of GBS and its variants have been published [55, 100–103].

Considering the interval between the onset of COVID-19 disease and symptoms of GBS and its variants, both para-infective and post-infective mechanisms have been postulated. An ongoing network among seven cities from northern Italy, in the epicenter of pandemic, is collecting data from patients with GBS diagnosed during the outbreak of SARS-CoV-2 infections.

References

1. Arbour N, Day R, Newcombe J, Talbot PJ. Neuroinvasion by human respiratory coronaviruses. J Virol. 2000;74:8913.
2. Desforges M, Le Coupanec A, Dubeau P, Bourgouin A, Lajoie L, Dubé M, Talbot PJ. Human coronaviruses and other respiratory viruses: underestimated opportunistic pathogens of the central nervous system? Viruses. 2019;12:14.
3. Verstrepen K, Baisier L, De Cauwer H. Neurological manifestations of COVID-19, SARS and MERS. Acta Neurol Belg. 2020;120:1051–60.
4. Lu R, Zhao X, Li J, et al. Genomic characterisation and epidemiology of 2019 novel coronavirus: implications for virus origins and receptor binding. Lancet. 2020;395:565–74.
5. Cao W, Li T. COVID-19: towards understanding of pathogenesis. Cell Res. 2020;30:367–9.

6. Li W, Moore MJ, Vasilieva N, et al. Angiotensin-converting enzyme 2 is a functional receptor for the SARS coronavirus. Nature. 2003;426:450–4.

7. Shang J, Ye G, Shi K, Wan Y, Luo C, Aihara H, Geng Q, Auerbach A, Li F. Structural basis of receptor recognition by SARS-CoV-2. Nature. 2020;581:221–4.

8. Rivellese F, Prediletto E. ACE2 at the centre of COVID-19 from paucisymptomatic infections to severe pneumonia. Autoimmun Rev. 2020;19:102536.

9. Hamming I, Timens W, Bulthuis MLC, Lely AT, Navis GJ, van Goor H. Tissue distribution of ACE2 protein, the functional receptor for SARS coronavirus. A first step in understanding SARS pathogenesis. J Pathol. 2004;203:631–7.

10. Sungnak W, Huang N, Bécavin C, et al. SARS-CoV-2 entry factors are highly expressed in nasal epithelial cells together with innate immune genes. Nat Med. 2020;26:681–7.

11. Xu Z, Shi L, Wang Y, et al. Pathological findings of COVID-19 associated with acute respiratory distress syndrome. Lancet Respir Med. 2020;8:420–2.

12. Zaim S, Chong JH, Sankaranarayanan V, Harky A. COVID-19 and multiorgan response. Curr Probl Cardiol. 2020;45:100618.

13. Puelles VG, Lütgehetmann M, Lindenmeyer MT, et al. Multiorgan and renal tropism of SARS-CoV-2. N Engl J Med. 2020;383:590–2.

14. Su H, Yang M, Wan C, et al. Renal histopathological analysis of 26 postmortem findings of patients with COVID-19 in China. Kidney Int. 2020;98:219–27.

15. Hanley B, Naresh KN, Roufosse C, et al. Histopathological findings and viral tropism in UK patients with severe fatal COVID-19: a post-mortem study. Lancet Microbe. 2020;1:e245–53.

16. Pedersen SF, Ho Y-C. SARS-CoV-2: a storm is raging. J Clin Invest. 2020;130:2202–5.

17. Jose RJ, Manuel A. COVID-19 cytokine storm: the interplay between inflammation and coagulation. Lancet Respir Med. 2020;8:e46–7.

18. Huang C, Wang Y, Li X. Clinical features of patients infected with 2019 novel coronavirus in Wuhan, China. Lancet. 2020;395:497.

19. RECOVERY Collaborative Group. Dexamethasone in hospitalized patients with covid-19—preliminary report. N Engl J Med. 2020; https://doi.org/10.1056/NEJMoa2021436.

20. Libby P, Lüscher T. COVID-19 is, in the end, an endothelial disease. Eur Heart J. 2020;41:3038–44.

21. Lowenstein CJ, Solomon SD. Severe COVID-19 is a microvascular disease. Circulation. 2020;142:1609. https://doi.org/10.1161/CIRCULATIONAHA.120.050354.

22. Teuwen L-A, Geldhof V, Pasut A, Carmeliet P. COVID-19: the vasculature unleashed. Nat Rev Immunol. 2020;20:389–91.

23. Varga Z, Flammer AJ, Steiger P, Haberecker M, Andermatt R, Zinkernagel AS, Mehra MR, Schuepbach RA, Ruschitzka F, Moch H. Endothelial cell infection and endotheliitis in COVID-19. Lancet. 2020;395:1417–8.

24. Magro C, Mulvey JJ, Berlin D, Nuovo G, Salvatore S, Harp J, Baxter-Stoltzfus A, Laurence J. Complement associated microvascular injury and thrombosis in the pathogenesis of severe COVID-19 infection: a report of five cases. Transl Res. 2020;220:1–13.

25. Rambaldi A, Gritti G, Micò MC, et al. Endothelial injury and thrombotic microangiopathy in COVID-19: treatment with the lectin-pathway inhibitor narsoplimab. Immunobiology. 2020;225:152001.

26. Kang S, Tanaka T, Inoue H, et al. IL-6 trans-signaling induces plasminogen activator inhibitor-1 from vascular endothelial cells in cytokine release syndrome. Proc Natl Acad Sci U S A. 2020;117:22351.

27. Kox M, Waalders NJB, Kooistra EJ, Gerretsen J, Pickkers P. Cytokine levels in critically ill patients with COVID-19 and other conditions. JAMA. 2020;324:1565–7.

28. Tsai L-K, Hsieh S-T, Chao C-C, Chen Y-C, Lin Y-H, Chang S-C, Chang Y-C. Neuromuscular disorders in severe acute respiratory syndrome. Arch Neurol. 2004;61:1669–73.

29. Chao CC, Tsai LK, Chiou YH, Tseng MT, Hsieh ST, Chang SC, Chang Y-C. Peripheral nerve disease in SARS. Neurology. 2003;61:1820.

30. Wang J-L, Wang J-T, Yu C-J, Chen Y-C, Hsueh P-R, Hsiao C-H, Kao C-L, Chang S-C, Yang P-C. Rhabdomyolysis associated with probable SARS. Am J Med. 2003;115:421–2.

31. Algahtani H, Subahi A, Shirah B. Neurological complications of middle east respiratory syndrome coronavirus: a report of two cases and review of the literature. Case Rep Neurol Med. 2016;2016:3502683.

32. Kim J-E, Heo J-H, Kim H, Song S, Park S-S, Park T-H, Ahn J-Y, Kim M-K, Choi J-P. Neurological complications during treatment of middle east respiratory syndrome. J Clin Neurol. 2017;13:227–33.

33. Umapathi T, Kor AC, Venketasubramanian N, et al. Large artery ischaemic stroke in severe acute respiratory syndrome (SARS). J Neurol. 2004;251:1227–31.

34. Arabi YM, Harthi A, Hussein J, et al. Severe neurologic syndrome associated with Middle East respiratory syndrome corona virus (MERS-CoV). Infection. 2015;43:495–501.

35. Mao L, Jin H, Wang M, et al. Neurologic manifestations of hospitalized patients with coronavirus disease 2019 in Wuhan, China. JAMA Neurol. 2020;77:683–90.

36. Karadaş Ö, Öztürk B, Sonkaya AR. A prospective clinical study of detailed neurological manifestations in patients with COVID-19. Neurol Sci. 2020;41:1991–5.

37. Helms J, Kremer S, Merdji H, et al. Neurologic features in severe SARS-CoV-2 infection. N Engl J Med. 2020;382:2268–70.

38. Paterson RW, Brown RL, Benjamin L, et al. The emerging spectrum of COVID-19 neurology: clinical, radiological and laboratory findings. Brain. 2020;143:3104.

39. Benussi A, Pilotto A, Premi E, et al. Clinical characteristics and outcomes of inpatients with neurologic

disease and COVID-19 in Brescia, Lombardy, Italy. Neurology. 2020;95:e910.

40. Varatharaj A, Thomas N, Ellul MA, et al. Neurological and neuropsychiatric complications of COVID-19 in 153 patients: a UK-wide surveillance study. Lancet Psychiatry. 2020;7:875.

41. Pinna P, Grewal P, Hall JP, et al. Neurological manifestations and COVID-19: experiences from a tertiary care center at the Frontline. J Neurol Sci. 2020;415:116969. https://doi.org/10.1016/j.jns.2020.116969.

42. Xiong W, Mu J, Guo J, et al. New onset neurologic events in people with COVID-19 in 3 regions in China. Neurology. 2020;95:e1479.

43. Rifino N, Censori B, Agazzi E, et al. Neurologic manifestations in 1760 COVID-19 patients admitted to Papa Giovanni XXIII Hospital, Bergamo, Italy. J Neurol. 2020:1–8. https://doi.org/10.1007/s00415-020-10251-5.

44. Bohmwald K, Gálvez NMS, Ríos M, Kalergis AM. Neurologic alterations due to respiratory virus infections. Front Cell Neurosci. 2018;12:386.

45. Baig AM, Khaleeq A, Ali U, Syeda H. Evidence of the COVID-19 virus targeting the CNS: tissue distribution, host–virus interaction, and proposed neurotropic mechanisms. ACS Chem Neurosci. 2020;11:995–8.

46. Netland J, Meyerholz DK, Moore S, Cassell M, Perlman S. Severe acute respiratory syndrome coronavirus infection causes neuronal death in the absence of encephalitis in mice transgenic for human ACE2. J Virol. 2008;82:7264.

47. Li K, Wohlford-Lenane C, Perlman S, Zhao J, Jewell AK, Reznikov LR, Gibson-Corley KN, Meyerholz DK, McCray PB Jr. Middle east respiratory syndrome coronavirus causes multiple organ damage and lethal disease in mice transgenic for human dipeptidyl peptidase 4. J Infect Dis. 2016;213:712–22.

48. Matsuda K, Park CH, Sunden Y, Kimura T, Ochiai K, Kida H, Umemura T. The vagus nerve is one route of transneural invasion for intranasally inoculated influenza A virus in mice. Vet Pathol. 2004;41:101–7.

49. Hadziefendic S, Haxhiu MA. CNS innervation of vagal preganglionic neurons controlling peripheral airways: a transneuronal labeling study using pseudorabies virus. J Auton Nerv Syst. 1999;76:135–45.

50. Morfopoulou S, Brown JR, Davies EG, et al. Human coronavirus OC43 associated with fatal encephalitis. N Engl J Med. 2016;375:497–8.

51. Hung ECW, Chim SSC, Chan PKS, Tong YK, Ng EKO, Chiu RWK, Leung C-B, Sung JJY, Tam JS, Lo YMD. Detection of SARS coronavirus RNA in the cerebrospinal fluid of a patient with severe acute respiratory syndrome. Clin Chem. 2003;49:2108–9.

52. Ding Y, He L, Zhang Q, et al. Organ distribution of severe acute respiratory syndrome (SARS) associated coronavirus (SARS-CoV) in SARS patients: implications for pathogenesis and virus transmission pathways. J Pathol. 2004;203:622–30.

53. Xu J, Zhong S, Liu J, et al. Detection of severe acute respiratory syndrome coronavirus in the brain: poten-

tial role of the chemokine mig in pathogenesis. Clin Infect Dis. 2005;41:1089–96.

54. Moriguchi T, Harii N, Goto J, et al. A first case of meningitis/encephalitis associated with SARS-Coronavirus-2. Int J Infect Dis. 2020;94:55–8.

55. Domingues RB, Mendes-Correa MC, de Moura Leite FBV, et al. First case of SARS-COV-2 sequencing in cerebrospinal fluid of a patient with suspected demyelinating disease. J Neurol. 2020;267:3154. https://doi.org/10.1007/s00415-020-09996-w.

56. Virhammar J, Kumlien E, Fällmar D, et al. Acute necrotizing encephalopathy with SARS-CoV-2 RNA confirmed in cerebrospinal fluid. Neurology. 2020;95:445.

57. Kremer S, Lersy F, de Sèze J, et al. Brain MRI findings in severe COVID-19: a retrospective observational study. Radiology. 2020;297:E242.

58. Schaller T, Hirschbühl K, Burkhardt K, Braun G, Trepel M, Märkl B, Claus R. Postmortem examination of patients with COVID-19. JAMA. 2020;323:2518–20.

59. Solomon IH, Normandin E, Bhattacharyya S, Mukerji SS, Keller K, Ali AS, Adams G, Hornick JL, Padera RF, Sabeti P. Neuropathological features of Covid-19. N Engl J Med. 2020;383:989–92.

60. Paniz-Mondolfi A, Bryce C, Grimes Z, Gordon RE, Reidy J, Lednicky J, Sordillo EM, Fowkes M. Central nervous system involvement by severe acute respiratory syndrome coronavirus-2 (SARS-CoV-2). J Med Virol. 2020;92:699–702.

61. Bikdeli B, Madhavan MV, Jimenez D, et al. COVID-19 and thrombotic or thromboembolic disease: implications for prevention, antithrombotic therapy, and follow-up: JACC state-of-the-art review. J Am Coll Cardiol. 2020;75:2950–73.

62. Zhang Y, Xiao M, Zhang S, et al. Coagulopathy and antiphospholipid antibodies in patients with Covid-19. N Engl J Med. 2020;382:e38.

63. Beyrouti R, Adams ME, Benjamin L, et al. Characteristics of ischaemic stroke associated with COVID-19. J Neurol Neurosurg Psychiatry. 2020;91:889.

64. Harzallah I, Debliquis A, Drénou B. Lupus anticoagulant is frequent in patients with Covid-19. J Thromb Haemost. 2020;18:2064–5.

65. Ackermann M, Verleden SE, Kuehnel M, et al. Pulmonary vascular endothelialitis, thrombosis, and angiogenesis in Covid-19. N Engl J Med. 2020;383:120–8.

66. Klok FA, Kruip MJHA, van der Meer NJM, et al. Incidence of thrombotic complications in critically ill ICU patients with COVID-19. Thromb Res. 2020;191:145–7.

67. Lodigiani C, Iapichino G, Carenzo L, et al. Venous and arterial thromboembolic complications in COVID-19 patients admitted to an academic hospital in Milan, Italy. Thromb Res. 2020;191:9–14.

68. Yaghi S, Ishida K, Torres J, et al. SARS-CoV-2 and stroke in a New York healthcare system. Stroke. 2020;51:2002–11.

69. Tan Y-K, Goh C, Leow AST, et al. COVID-19 and ischemic stroke: a systematic review and meta-summary of the literature. J Thromb Thrombolysis. 2020;50:587–95.

70. George N, Patrik M, Georgios G, et al. Characteristics and outcomes in patients with COVID-19 and acute ischemic stroke. Stroke. 2020;51:e254–8.

71. McIntosh K. Coronavirus disease 2019 (covid-19): clinical features. 2020. https://www.Uptodate.Com/contents/coronavirus-disease-2019-covid-19-clinical-features. Accessed 18 Jun 2020.

72. Wang A, Mandigo GK, Yim PD, Meyers PM, Lavine SD. Stroke and mechanical thrombectomy in patients with COVID-19: technical observations and patient characteristics. J Neurointervent Surg. 2020;12:648.

73. Oxley TJ, Mocco J, Majidi S, et al. Large-vessel stroke as a presenting feature of Covid-19 in the young. N Engl J Med. 2020;382:e60.

74. Dogra S, Jain R, Cao M, et al. Hemorrhagic stroke and anticoagulation in COVID-19. J Stroke Cerebrovasc Dis. 2020;29:104984. https://doi.org/10.1016/j.jstrokecerebrovasdis.2020.104984.

75. Hoelscher C, Sweid A, Ghosh R, et al. Cerebral deep venous thrombosis and COVID-19: case report. J Neurosurg. 2020:1–4.

76. Garaci F, Di Giuliano F, Picchi E, Da Ros V, Floris R. Venous cerebral thrombosis in COVID-19 patient. J Neurol Sci. 2020;414:116871.

77. Malentacchi M, Gned D, Angelino V, Demichelis S, Perboni A, Veltri A, Bertolotto A, Capobianco M. Concomitant brain arterial and venous thrombosis in a COVID-19 patient. Eur J Neurol. 2020;27:e38–9.

78. Romero-Sánchez CM, Díaz-Maroto I, Fernández-Díaz E, et al. Neurologic manifestations in hospitalized patients with COVID-19. Neurology. 2020;95:e1060.

79. Duong L, Xu P, Liu A. Meningoencephalitis without respiratory failure in a young female patient with COVID-19 infection in Downtown Los Angeles, early April 2020. Brain Behav Immun. 2020;87:33.

80. Huang YH, Jiang D, Huang JT. SARS-CoV-2 detected in cerebrospinal fluid by PCR in a case of COVID-19 encephalitis. Brain Behav Immun. 2020;87:149.

81. Bernard-Valnet R, Pizzarotti B, Anichini A, Demars Y, Russo E, Schmidhauser M, Cerutti-Sola J, Rossetti AO, Du Pasquier R. Two patients with acute meningoencephalitis concomitant with SARS-CoV-2 infection. Eur J Neurol. 2020;27:e43–4.

82. Pilotto A, Odolini S, Masciocchi S, et al. Steroid-responsive encephalitis in coronavirus disease 2019. Ann Neurol. 2020;88:423–7.

83. Dogan L, Kaya D, Sarikaya T, Zengin R, Dincer A, Akinci IO, Afsar N. Plasmapheresis treatment in COVID-19-related autoimmune meningoencephalitis: case series. Brain Behav Immun. 2020;87:155–8.

84. Poyiadji N, Shahin G, Noujaim D, Stone M, Patel S, Griffith B. COVID-19–associated acute hemorrhagic necrotizing encephalopathy: imaging features. Radiology. 2020;296:E119–20.

85. Dixon L, Varley J, Gontsarova A, et al. COVID-19-related acute necrotizing encephalopathy with brain stem involvement in a patient with aplastic anemia. Neurol Neuroimmunol Neuroinflamm. 2020;7:e789.

86. Pilotto A, Masciocchi S, Volonghi I, et al. Clinical presentation and outcomes of SARS-CoV-2 related encephalitis: the ENCOVID multicentre study. J Infect Dis. 2020;223:28.

87. Abdelhady M, Elsotouhy A, Vattoth S. Acute flaccid myelitis in COVID-19. BJR Case Rep. 2020;6:20200098.

88. AlKetbi R, AlNuaimi D, AlMulla M, AlTalai N, Samir M, Kumar N, AlBastaki U. Acute myelitis as a neurological complication of Covid-19: a case report and MRI findings. Radiol Case Rep. 2020;15:1591–5.

89. Chow CCN, Magnussen J, Ip J, Su Y. Acute transverse myelitis in COVID-19 infection. BMJ Case Rep. 2020;13:e236720.

90. Munz M, Wessendorf S, Koretsis G, Tewald F, Baegi R, Krämer S, Geissler M, Reinhard M. Acute transverse myelitis after COVID-19 pneumonia. J Neurol. 2020;267:2196–7.

91. Sotoca J, Rodríguez-Álvarez Y. COVID-19-associated acute necrotizing myelitis. Neurol Neuroimmunol Neuroinflamm. 2020;7:e803.

92. Zhao K, Huang J, Dai D, Feng Y, Liu L, Nie S. Acute myelitis after SARS-CoV-2 infection: a case report. medRxiv. 2020; https://doi.org/10.1101/2020.03.16.20035105.

93. Maideniuc C, Memon AB. Acute necrotizing myelitis and acute motor axonal neuropathy in a COVID-19 patient. J Neurol. 2020:1–3.

94. Masuccio FG, Barra M, Claudio G, Claudio S. A rare case of acute motor axonal neuropathy and myelitis related to SARS-CoV-2 infection. J Neurol. 2020:1–4. https://doi.org/10.1007/s00415-020-10219-5.

95. Zhou S, Jones-Lopez EC, Soneji DJ, Azevedo CJ, Patel VR. Myelin oligodendrocyte glycoprotein antibody-associated optic neuritis and myelitis in COVID-19. J Neuroophthalmol. 2020;40:398–402.

96. Ibekwe TS, Fasunla AJ, Orimadegun AE. Systematic review and meta-analysis of smell and taste disorders in COVID-19. OTO Open. 2020;4:2473974X20957975.

97. Zhao H, Shen D, Zhou H, Liu J, Chen S. Guillain-Barré syndrome associated with SARS-CoV-2 infection: causality or coincidence? Lancet Neurol. 2020;19:383–4.

98. Alberti P, Beretta S, Piatti M, et al. Guillain-Barré syndrome related to COVID-19 infection. Neurol Neuroimmunol Neuroinflamm. 2020;7:e741.

99. Toscano G, Palmerini F, Ravaglia S, et al. Guillain–Barré syndrome associated with SARS-CoV-2. N Engl J Med. 2020;382:2574–6.

100. Lantos JE, Strauss SB, Lin E. COVID-19–associated miller fisher syndrome: MRI findings. AJNR Am J Neuroradiol. 2020;41:1184. https://doi.org/10.3174/ajnr.A6609.

101. Manganotti P, Pesavento V, Buoite Stella A, Bonzi L, Campagnolo E, Bellavita G, Fabris B, Luzzati R. Miller Fisher syndrome diagnosis and treatment in a patient with SARS-CoV-2. J Neurovirol. 2020;26:605–6.

102. Reyes-Bueno JA, García-Trujillo L, Urbaneja P, Ciano-Petersen NL, Postigo-Pozo MJ, Martínez-Tomás C, Serrano-Castro PJ. Miller-Fisher syndrome after SARS-CoV-2 infection. Eur J Neurol. 2020;27:1759–61.

103. Assini A, Benedetti L, Di Maio S, Schirinzi E, Del Sette M. New clinical manifestation of COVID-19 related Guillain-Barrè syndrome highly responsive to intravenous immunoglobulins: two Italian cases. Neurol Sci. 2020;41:1657–8.

Vascular Manifestations in COVID 19

Antonino Barletta, Maria Luisa Colleoni,
Luca Quilici, Gabriele Gallizioli,
and Simonetta Gerevini

Neurological symptoms described in COVID-19 infected patients (hypo-ageusia, anosmia, confusion, seizures, etc.) are often associated to presence of stroke and/or brain hemorrhages that sometimes can occur together. As COVID-19 has spread around the world, evidence has grown for an association with cerebrovascular disease. The association between COVID-19 and cerebrovascular complications were reported in an early retrospective case series from Wuhan [1], Italy [2, 3], and Netherlands [4] and extensively reported in Chap. 2.

The reported incidence of cerebrovascular disease in patients testing positive for SARS-CoV-2 ranges from 1% to 6%, potentially equating to large numbers of individuals as the pandemic progresses in some countries [5, 6], and multiple regions with high COVID-19 prevalence have reported stable or increased incidence of large vessel stroke and increased incidence of cryptogenic stroke (patients with no found typical cause of stroke).

Moreover the mean patient age in several thrombectomy case series of COVID-19 is younger than the typical population having this procedure [7–9], and case-control analysis of acute stroke protocol imaging from late March to early April, 2020, across a large New York City health system showed that, after adjusting for age, sex, and vascular risk factors, SAS-CoV-2 positivity was independently associated with stroke.

Some hypotheses have been postulated to explain cerebrovascular involvement in this infection.

The ACE1-Angiotensin II system is more active in the elderly males and this might explain why increasing mortality and cerebrovascular complications are observed more often in these patients [10, 11].

Early indicators suggest that another process linked with these cerebrovascular complications is the onset of a sepsis-induced coagulopathy (SIC), precursor of disseminated intravascular coagulation (DIC), due to an uncontrolled cytokine release [12]. Endothelial damage and thrombogenic-hemorrhagic processes are compounded by SARS-COV2 neurotropic and neuro invasive ability [13], demonstrated on other strains of human coronavirus in the past [14]. The alteration of coagulability resulted confirmed by the effectiveness of anticoagulant therapy with heparin or rTPA [15].

Lower levels of lymphocytes, platelet count, and higher blood urea nitrogen were also found in patients with CNS symptoms. No laboratory

A. Barletta · M. L. Colleoni · L. Quilici · G. Gallizioli
S. Gerevini (✉)
Neuroradiology Department, Papa Giovanni XXIII
Hospital, Bergamo, Italy
e-mail: abarletta@asst-pg23.it;
mcolleoni@asst-pg23.it; lquilici@asst-pg23.it;
ggallizioli@asst-pg23.it; sgerevini@asst-pg23.it

differences were found between patients with stroke or cerebral hemorrhage.

From an imaging point of view, no peculiar aspects, helpful to discriminate cerebrovascular complications of COVID-19 from classical stroke clinical presentation, were reported at the moment.

Therefore, for this reason arterial and venous imaging evaluation is essential for COVID-19 patients with acute cerebrovascular events, keeping in mind that data supporting an association between COVID-19 and stroke in young populations without typical vascular risk factors, at times with only mild respiratory symptoms, are increasing.

Numerous studies in the literature have investigated the correlation between stroke and cardiovascular and inflammatory events during COVID-19 infection.

Cardiac involvement with acute cardiac injury, arrhythmias and heart failure in COVID-19 patients has been described [16–18]. A meta-analysis of six studies observed cardiac injury in 8.0% patients, mostly occurring in patients who were sicker and in the ICU [19]. The hypothesized mechanisms, including an acute inflammatory response and plaque destabilization, could potentially lead to a cardioembolic stroke.

The relationship between inflammation and stroke is complex because the inflammation could precede, causing it, the stroke, or follow it [20, 21]. The interaction between inflammatory cells within the vascular wall and conventional risk factors alters the dynamics of atherosclerosis. This has a potential to acutely worsen in the presence of systemic inflammation and effect the coagulation cascade [22, 23].

In reference to risk factors the literature data suggest age and comorbidities like hypertension, diabetes and cardiovascular disease to be associated with higher mortality in COVID-19 [18, 24, 25]. In particular a report of patients with COVID-19 and stroke emphasizes coexistence of history of smoking (38.5%), alcohol intake (15.4%), and increased blood pressure (≥130/80 mmHg) (53.8%) [26].

Moreover, patients with stroke were more likely to have other underlying disorders, including hypertension (69.2% vs. 22.1%, $p < 0.001$) and diabetes mellitus (46.2% vs. 12.0%, $p < 0.01$) [28]. A report from the Chinese Center for Disease Control and Prevention describes a significantly higher mortality rate in patients with hypertension, diabetes and CVD (6%, 7.3% and 10.5%, respectively, versus an overall rate of 2.5%) among 44,672 COVID-19 cases. Some more details about cardiac involvement will be summarized in Chap. 6 (Other possible location of Cov-19 infection).

From an interventional neuroradiological point of view, the treatment of stroke does not differ based on the presence or absence of COVID-19 infection.

However, stroke management can be challenging as it involves the need to harmonize the "time is brain" concept and the safe and effective management of the potential spreading source of the virus. The triage processes during needs to ascertain whether the patient is a COVID suspect and delineate pathways for timely treatment and minimum exposure to health care personnel. The organization and management of the out-of-hospital territorial emergency must consider both the number of confirmed infections and the organizational capacity of structures not ready to manage stroke. Similarly, the hospital organization will have to consider adequate logistical and structural changes. Guidelines to manage patients with acute stroke during COVID-19 have been published [27, 28], giving more and more importance to the concept of "protected stroke code."

As discussed above, one of the supposed pathogenetic mechanisms in COVID viral infection is coagulopathy induced by a proinflammatory state.

This aspect should be considered when dealing with hemorrhagic manifestations of stroke. Discussions regarding anticoagulation for COVID-19 patients have been intensifying as evidence of hypercoagulability in this population continues to accumulate. Recent literature findings can be helpful in this regard. In a cohort of 755 patients diagnosed with positive COVID-19 and with neuroimaging, 4.4% had ICH [29]. The majority of these patients received therapeutic anticoagulation, most commonly UFH. The most frequent indication for starting anticoagulation was elevated D-dimer levels, reflecting what is indicated by the literature data.

In our center, from March to May 2020, we evaluated a cohort of 205 COVID+ patients. All underwent at least one brain CT. Forty-five underwent a brain CT angiography and 50 a brain MRI (50% of these on 3 T Magnet). Forty percent (79/205) of the brain CTs showed pathological changes; in particular among these 33% showed lobar infarcts, 37% lacunar infarct, and 35% hemorrhagic stroke. On MRI we registered a recurrent pattern of ischemic and/or haemorrhagic lesions in 50% of patients.

3.1   Clinical Cases

Case 1 F, 63 years old. Acute onset of severe dyspnea associated with confusion, diplopia and speech difficulties. In the previous days she reported fever and flu-like symptoms. FpO$_2$ values between 85% and 89% (Figs. 3.1, 3.2, 3.3, 3.4, 3.5, 3.6, 3.7, and 3.8).

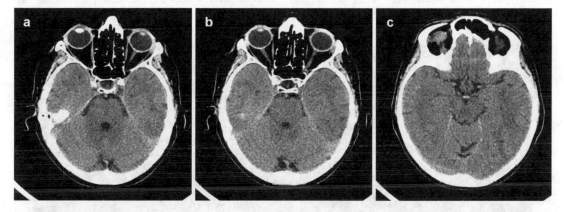

Fig. 3.1 Axial CT scan images show a point-like hyperdensity at the apex of the basilar artery. The tomodensitometric values in the posterior cranial fossa do not show alterations of suspected acute ischemic or hemorrhagic significance

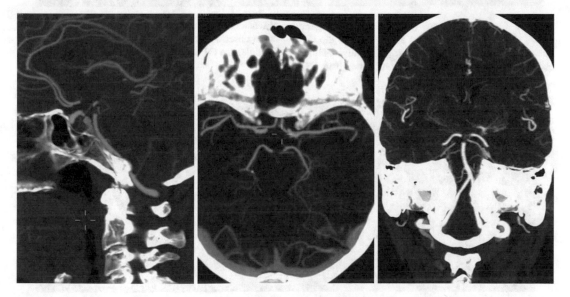

Fig. 3.2 CT angiography study. Multiplanar MIP reconstructions show thromboembolic defect at the apex of the basilar artery in sagittal, axial and coronal planes. The opacification defect involves the P1 tract of the posterior cerebral arteries and the emergence of the superior cerebellar arteries

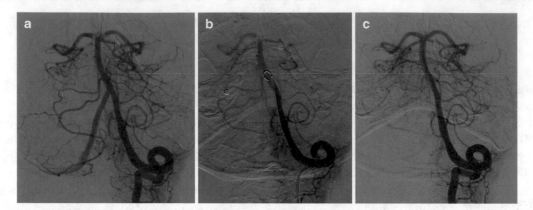

Fig. 3.3 Digital subtraction angiography. Superselective catheterization of the left vertebro-basilar arterial axis demonstrates and confirms the thromboembolic defect at the apex of the basilar artery (**a**, **b**). The mechanical thrombectomy procedure led to recanalization of the arterial axes (**c**)

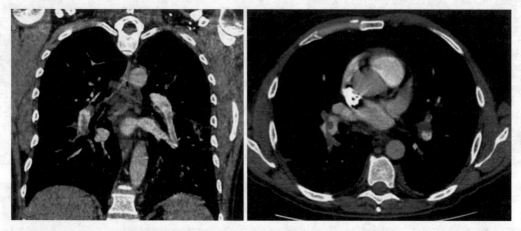

Fig. 3.4 Contrast enhanced chest CT. The investigation shows multiple filling defects at the level of the main branches of the pulmonary arteries, bilaterally. Findings compatible with pulmonary thromboembolism. The absence of dilation of the right heart cavities suggests an acute onset. After 24 h, due to the sudden onset of left hemiplegia a CT scan is performed

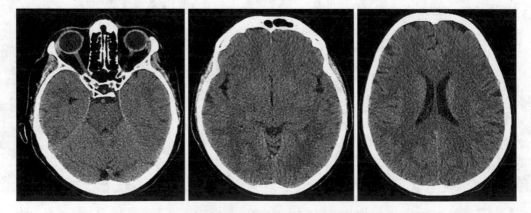

Fig. 3.5 Axial CT scan does not show tomodensitometric changes referable to ischemic or hemorrhagic lesions. There is only a slight minor representation of the cortical sulci on the left

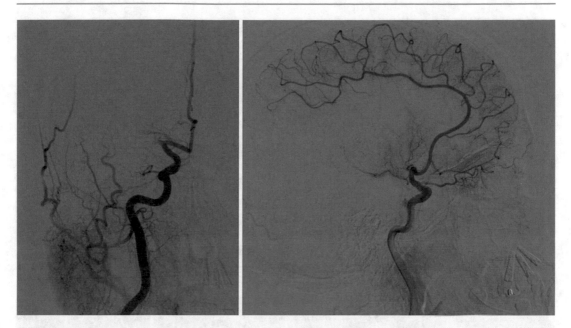

Fig. 3.6 Digital subtraction angiography. Super selective catheterization of the left internal carotid artery demonstrates complete occlusion of the middle cerebral artery at the M1 segment. The thromboembolic defect causes the complete absence of the cerebral parenchymography of the corresponding vascular territory, with evidence of retrograde opacification of the ipsilateral external carotid

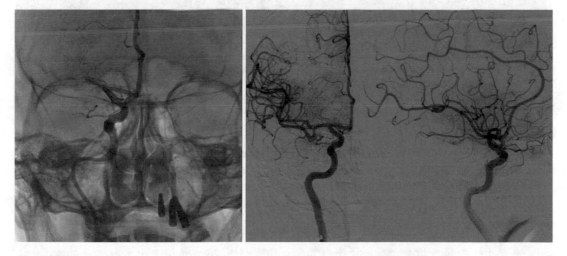

Fig. 3.7 Digital subtraction angiography. Two attempts of recanalization through mechanical thrombectomy lead to the revascularization of the vascular territory downstream of the previously highlighted refilling defect

Case 2 Male, 61 years old Dyspnea and fever for 5 days; presenting with dysarthria. SWAB+; Chest CT+ (Fig. 3.9).

Upon arrival in the emergency room, relatives report behavioral changes in the previous days (Figs. 3.10, 3.11, and 3.12).

Case 3 M, 55 years old. Rapid onset of acute headache associated with right hemi syndrome.

Case 4 M, 63 years old. Gradual onset of headache. Patient arrives to the emergency room on his

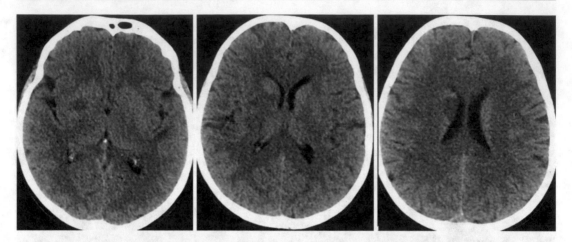

Fig. 3.8 Excellent clinical outcome (90 days mRs = 1). Ischemic hypodensity of right lenticular nucleus, right capsula interna and ipsilateral nuclei caudate. Mild mass effect on the right lateral ventricle with no midline shift

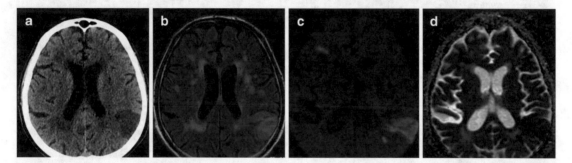

Fig. 3.9 Axial CT scan (**a**) shows a focal hypodensity in the left posterior parietal area. The periventricular white matter appears diffusely hypodense, due to advanced vascular disease. However, in the right anterior periventricular site, a further more focal reduction of tomodensitometric values is documented. Axial MRI FLAIR (**b**) highlights a focal left posterior parietal hyperintensity. Additional hyperintensity foci are associated, especially in the contralateral anterior periventricular site. There is a strong DWI and ADC correlation in these locations (**c, d**)

own after about 2 days of symptoms. Fever and mild dyspnea are associated, with FpO$_2$ values between 95% and 97% (Figs. 3.13, 3.14, and 3.15).

Case 5 F, 69 years old. The patient is taken to the emergency room by an advanced rescue vehicle due to the sudden appearance of dysarthria and dizziness (Figs. 3.16, 3.17, 3.18, and 3.19).

Case 6 F, 62 years old. Recent history of hospitalization for fever and dyspnea. Finding of COVID-19 related pneumonia. Following onset of unclear neurological symptoms, brain CT is performed (Figs. 3.20, 3.21, 3.22, and 3.23).

Case 6: ex-post re-interpretation: the lack of complete clinical information due to the peculiar moment of the pandemic, the execution of the first CT scan not in the proper acute phase of the neurological symptoms made difficult the correct definition and classification of this case. As a matter of fact, the actual revision of imaging opens a differential diagnostic issue versus PRES or PRES like classification. We consider this case here as a "vascular" case because it has been classified and treated as vascular; furthermore, we are conscious of possible different interpretations such as PRES like lesion.

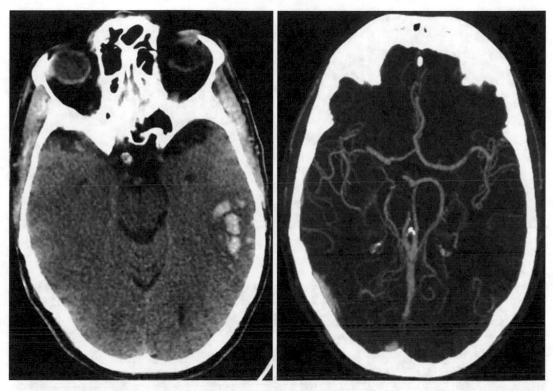

Fig. 3.10 Axial CT scan image (on right) and axial angio-CT scan image with MIP reconstruction (on the left) show temporal hemorrhagic lesion with no vascular ischemic alteration on the CT angiogram This kind of hemorrhage is atypical for location in absence of any vascular pathological findings

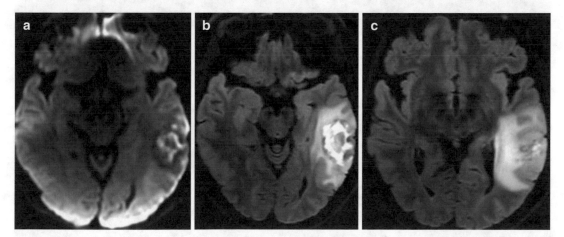

Fig. 3.11 Axial MRI. DWI (*b*-value: 1000) shows restriction into left temporal hemorrhagic lesion with surrounding edema (**a**) with a correlated ADC map showing restriction into left temporal hemorrhagic lesion with surrounding edema (**d**). **Axial FLAIR** (**b**, **c**) and **Axial T2w** (**e**) show left temporal hemorrhagic lesion with peripheral edema. (**f**) **Axial SWI**. Left temporal hemorrhagic lesion. Widespread hypointense changes can be seen at the site of the lesion. This finding is suggestive for the presence of hemosiderin deposits deriving from hemoglobin catabolism and from slow blood flow

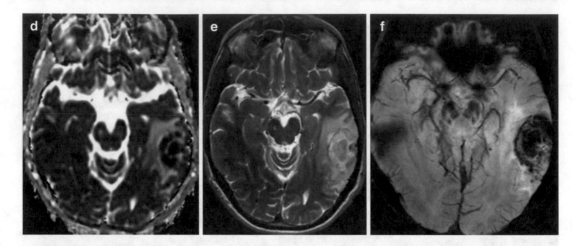

Fig. 3.11 (continued)

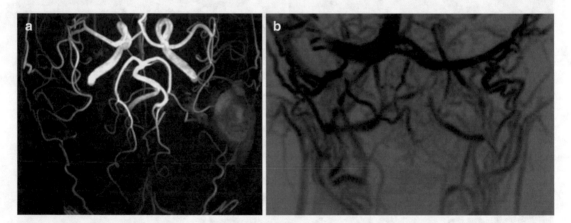

Fig. 3.12 Angio 3D Tof MIP reconstruction (**a**) shows no vascular malformations or lesions. Venous phase angio MRI (**b**): Left sigmoid sinus thrombosis

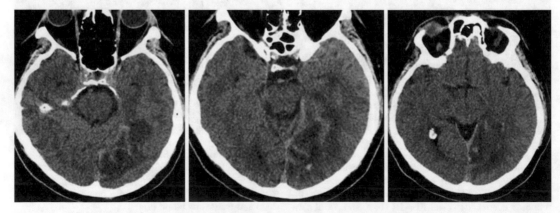

Fig. 3.13 Axial CT scan images show temporo-occipital hypodense lesions with hyperdense hemorrhagic alterations and perilesional edema. These findings are compat- ible with hemorrhagic transformation of the ischemic lesion. Uncertain ischemic hypodensity is also visible at the temporal and occipital-parietal right lobes

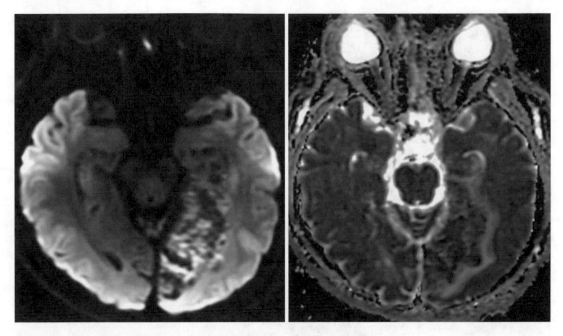

Fig. 3.14 Axial MRI. DWI (*b*-value: 1000) shows inhomogeneous hyperintense left temporo-occipital area of restricted diffusion. This finding is correlated with hypointensity ADC map

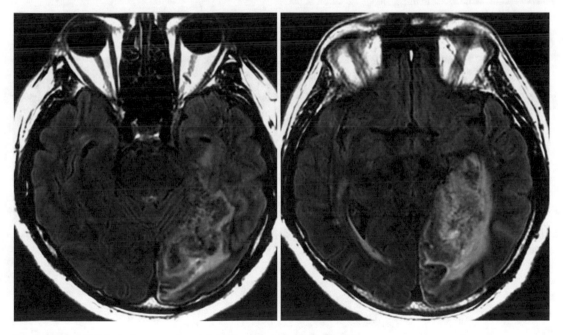

Fig. 3.15 Axial Flair. Left temporal\occipital inhomogeneous ischemic lesion

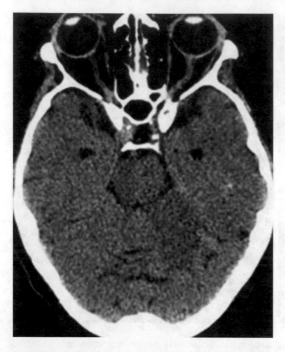

Fig. 3.16 Axial CT scan image shows ischemic hypodensity at the superior part of the left cerebellar hemisphere, SCA vascular territory, with dimensional reduction of the cerebellopontine cistern due to conspicuous perilesional edema

Case 7 F, 77 years old. Right hemiparesis. Fever and dyspnea of mild onset rapidly progressing are associated (Fig. 3.24).

Case 8 F, 82 years old. History of previous ischemic stroke. Acute appearance of aphasia and confusion. Fever and severe dyspnea (Figs. 3.25 and 3.26).

Case 9 M, 67 years old. Very rapid onset of severe dyspnea associated to Progressive neurological deterioration and coma (Figs. 3.27 and 3.28).

Case 10 M, 66 years old. Acute right hemi syndrome dx: during the various attempts at thrombectomy, thrombi continue to be created due to the state of hypercoagulation make the procedure really difficult (Figs. 3.29, 3.30, 3.31, 3.32, 3.33, and 3.34).

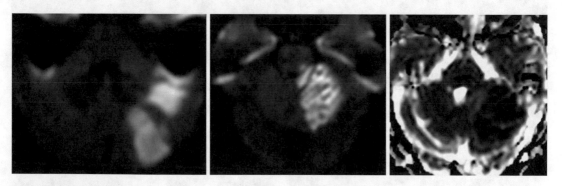

Fig. 3.17 Axial MRI. DWI (*b*-value: 1000) shows restriction at the superior part of the left cerebellar hemisphere, SCA vascular territory with a correlated ADC map

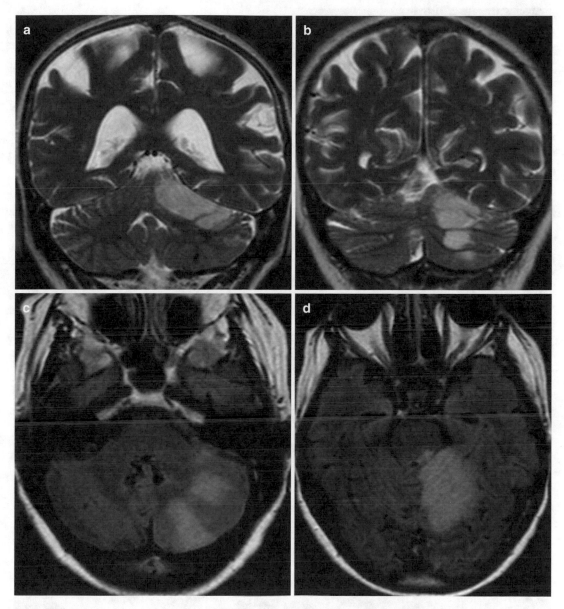

Fig. 3.18 Coronal T2w scan. Hyperintensity of the superior cerebellar hemisphere (**a**, **b**). Axial FLAIR (**c**, **d**) shows a perfect overlap of anomalous signal hyperintensity

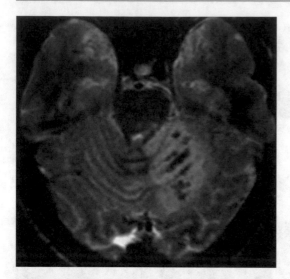

Fig. 3.19 Axial T2*w. The "blooming effect" in the context of the cerebellar lesion is highlighted

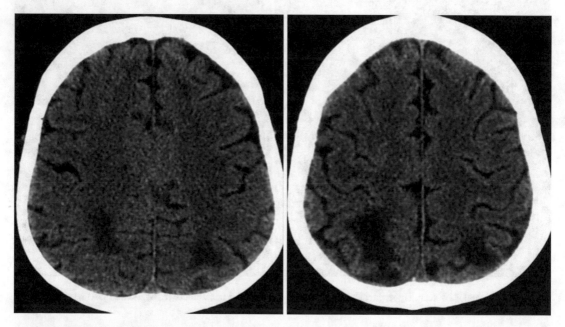

Fig. 3.20 Axial CT scan images show cortical-subcortical hypodensity in both parietal lobes with no hemorrhagic lesions. Findings were defined as compatible with bilateral ischemic lesions

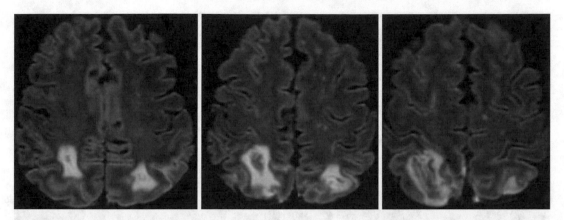

Fig. 3.21 Axial FLAIR shows hyperintense biparietal quite symmetrical lesions predominantly in subcortical region

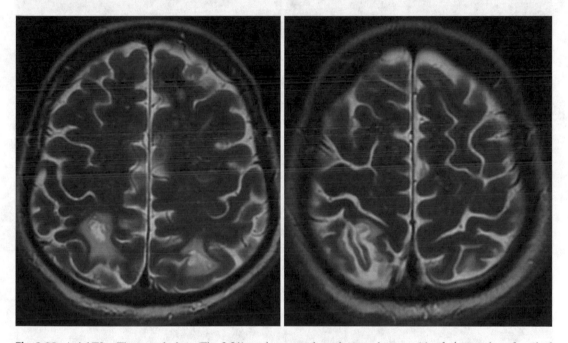

Fig. 3.22 Axial T2w. The same lesions (Fig. 3.21) can be seen as hyperintense changes with relative sparing of cortical regions. No further alterations of suspected ischemic significance are detectable

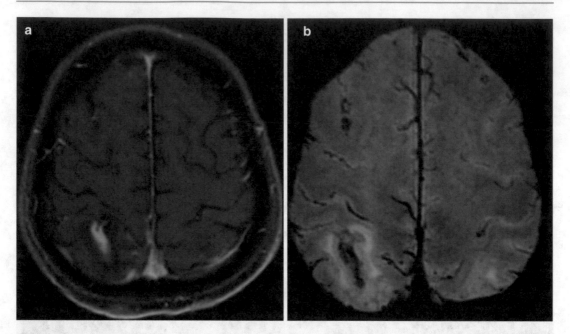

Fig. 3.23 Axial contrast enhanced T1w (**a**) shows a brilliant "gyral" enhancement associated to a focal T2* hypo intensity (**b**) suggestive for the presence of hemosiderin deposits deriving from hemoglobin catabolism

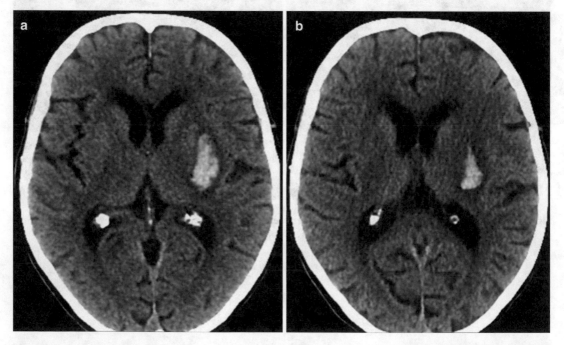

Fig. 3.24 Axial CT scan (**a**, **b**) shows the presence of left nucleus-capsular hematoma associated with a conspicuous area of peri lesional edema. (**c**) The finding is associated with chest X-ray showing the presence of signs referable to accentuation of the interstitial texture in a patient with a clinical suggestive of COVID-19 related interstitial pneumonia

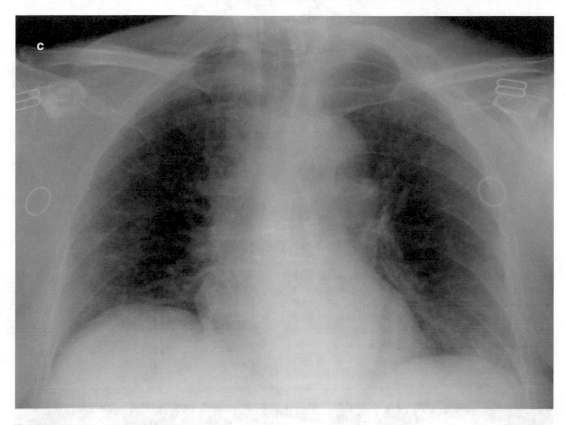

Fig. 3.24 (continued)

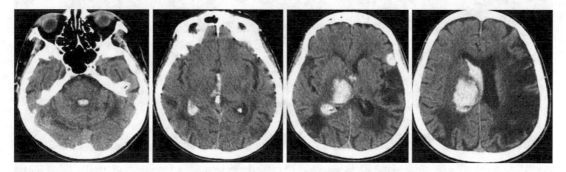

Fig. 3.25 Axial CT scan shows right capsule-thalamic-lenticular hemorrhagic collection, with minimal perilesional edema and blood flooding of the right lateral ventricle, of the third and fourth ventricles. Left deviation of the pellucid septum. Concomitant presence of extensive hemispheric infarct outcomes on the left

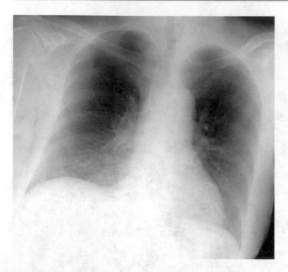

Fig. 3.26 Chest X-ray showing the presence of signs referable to accentuation of the interstitial texture in a patient with a clinical suggestive of COVID-19 related interstitial pneumonia. There is no evidence of focal parenchymal thickening or signs uniquely referable to volume overload of the pulmonary circulation

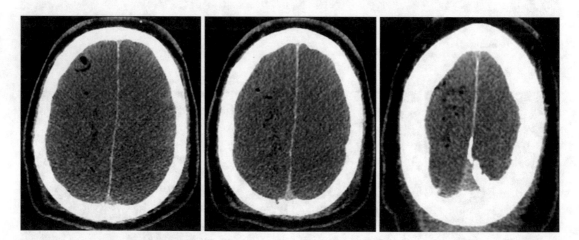

Fig. 3.27 Axial CT scan shows a diffuse supratentorial cerebral edema and diffuse cerebral parenchymal hypodensity. There is cortical sulci effacement and the difference between white and gray matter is no longer present. The presence of intraparenchymal aerial components of unknown etiology is highlighted

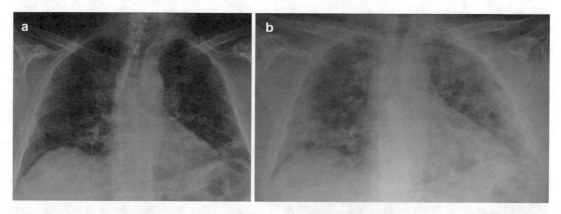

Fig. 3.28 Serial chest X-ray (**a**) shows worsening of the pulmonary radiographic picture with the appearance (**b**) of accentuation of the interstitial texture in a patient with a clinical suggestive of COVID-19 related interstitial pneumonia. The relief is also associated with the appearance of more compact parenchymal thickening in the right lung and reduced lung capacity

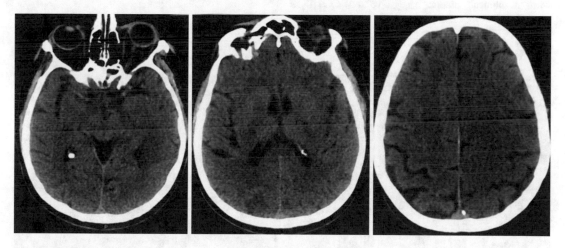

Fig. 3.29 Axial CT scan (**a**) image show point-like hyperdense left proximal middle cerebral artery (M1-M2 segment). Axial CT scan images (**b**, **c**) shows low density area effacing left insular ribbon and slight minor representation of the cortical sulci on the left

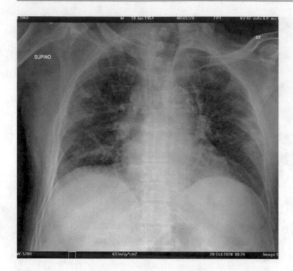

Fig. 3.30 Chest X-ray showing radiological signs referable to accentuation of the interstitial texture in a patient with a clinical picture suggestive of COVID-19 pneumonia

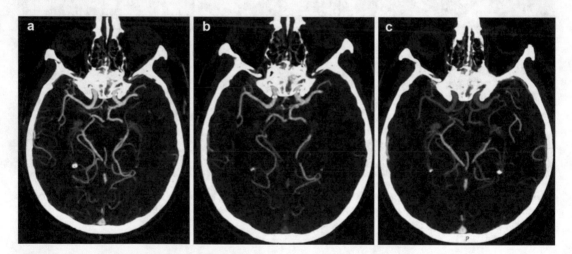

Fig. 3.31 CT angiography multiphase study; MIP reconstructions show the thromboembolic defect at left proximal cerebral (M1-M2) medial artery (**a**, **b**); and bad collateralization; avascular fronto-temporal area in the late fase of CT angiogram (**b**, **c**)

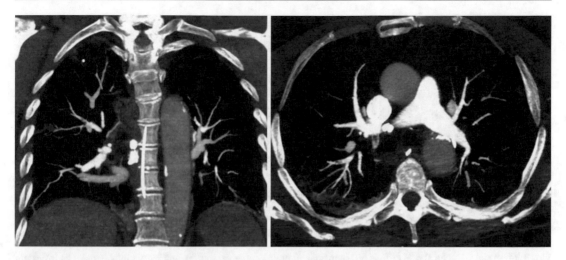

Fig. 3.32 Contrast enhanced chest CT. The investigation shows the presence of multiple filling defects at the level of the secondary branches of the right pulmonary arteries. Findings compatible with pulmonary thromboembolism

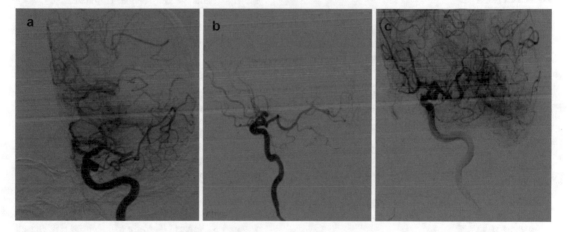

Fig. 3.33 Digital subtraction angiography. Super selective catheterization of the left internal carotid artery demonstrates occlusion of the middle cerebral artery at the M2 segment (**a**). The thromboembolic defect causes the complete absence of the cerebral parenchymography of the corresponding vascular territory (**b**) and (**c**) images with occlusion also the distal (A2-A3 segment) left anterior cerebral artery. Multiple successive attempts of recanalization through mechanical thrombectomy failed

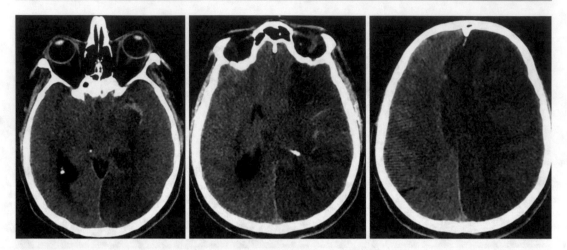

Fig. 3.34 Axial CT scan shows diffuse left hemispheric brain edema-cerebral parenchymal hypodensity as for extensive left infarct in middle and anterior cerebral artery's territories

References

1. Mao L, Jin H, Wang M, et al. Neurologic manifestations of hospitalized patients with coronavirus disease 2019 in Wuhan, China. JAMA Neurol. 2020;77:683–90.
2. Lodigiani C, Iapichino G, Carenzo L, et al. Venous and arterial thromboembolic complications in COVID-19 patients admitted to an academic hospital in Milan, Italy. Thromb Res. 2020;191:9–14.
3. Benussi A, Pilotto A, Premi E, et al. Clinical characteristics and outcomes of inpatients with neurologic disease and COVID-19 in Brescia, Lombardy. Neurology. 2020;95:e910.
4. Klok FA, Kruip MJHA, van der Meer NJM, et al. Incidence of thrombotic complications in critically ill ICU patients with COVID-19. Thromb Res. 2020;191:145–7.
5. Ellul MA, Benjamin L, Singh B, Lant S, Michael BD, Easton A, Kneen R, Defres S, Sejvar J, Solomon T. Neurological associations of COVID-19. Lancet Neurol. 2020;19:767–83.
6. Merkler AE, Parikh NS, Mir S, et al. Risk of ischemic stroke in patients with Covid-19 versus patients with influenza. medRxiv. 2020; https://doi.org/10.1101/2020.05.18.20105494.
7. Wang A, Mandigo GK, Yim PD, Meyers PM, Lavine SD. Stroke and mechanical thrombectomy in patients with COVID-19: technical observations and patient characteristics. J Neurointervent Surg. 2020;12:648.
8. Simon E, Benjamin M, Hocine R, et al. Treatment of acute ischemic stroke due to large vessel occlusion with COVID-19. Stroke. 2020;51:2540–3.
9. Sweid A, Hammoud B, Bekelis K, et al. Cerebral ischemic and hemorrhagic complications of coronavirus disease 2019. Int J Stroke. 2020;15:733–42.
10. Xudong X, Junzhu C, Xingxiang W, Furong Z, Yanrong L. Age- and gender-related difference of ACE2 expression in rat lung. Life Sci. 2006;78:2166–71.
11. Wang M, Monticone RE, Lakatta EG. Proinflammation of aging central arteries: a mini-review. Gerontology. 2014;60:519–29.
12. Poyiadji N, Cormier P, Patel PY, et al. Acute pulmonary embolism and COVID-19. Radiology. 2020;297:E335.
13. Arbour N, Day R, Newcombe J, Talbot PJ. Neuroinvasion by human respiratory coronaviruses. J Virol. 2000;74:8913.
14. Desforges M, Le Coupanec A, Brison E, Meessen-Pinard M, Talbot PJ. Neuroinvasive and neurotropic human respiratory coronaviruses: potential neurovirulent agents in humans. Adv Exp Med Biol. 2014;807:75–96.
15. Wang J, Hajizadeh N, Moore EE, McIntyre RC, Moore PK, Veress LA, Yaffe MB, Moore HB, Barrett CD. Tissue plasminogen activator (tPA) treatment for COVID-19 associated acute respiratory distress syndrome (ARDS): a case series. J Thromb Haemost. 2020;18:1752–5.
16. Guo T, Fan Y, Chen M, Wu X, Zhang L, He T, Wang H, Wan J, Wang X, Lu Z. Cardiovascular implications of fatal outcomes of patients with coronavirus disease 2019 (COVID-19). JAMA Cardiol. 2020;5:811–8.
17. Bansal M. Cardiovascular disease and COVID-19. Diabetes Metab Synd. 2020;14:247–50.
18. Wang D, Hu B, Hu C, et al. Clinical characteristics of 138 hospitalized patients with 2019 novel coronavirus-infected pneumonia in Wuhan, China. JAMA. 2020;323:1061–9.
19. Li B, Yang J, Zhao F, Zhi L, Wang X, Liu L, Bi Z, Zhao Y. Prevalence and impact of cardiovascular metabolic diseases on COVID-19 in China. Clin Res Cardiol. 2020;109:531–8.

20. Lindsberg PJ, Grau AJ. Inflammation and infections as risk factors for ischemic stroke. Stroke. 2003;34:2518–32.

21. Shi K, Tian D-C, Li Z-G, Ducruet AF, Lawton MT, Shi F-D. Global brain inflammation in stroke. Lancet Neurol. 2019;18:1058–66.

22. Arenillas Juan F, José Á-S, Molina Carlos A, Pilar C, Joan M, Álex R, Bernardo I, Manuel Q. C-reactive protein predicts further ischemic events in first-ever transient ischemic attack or stroke patients with intracranial large-artery occlusive disease. Stroke. 2003;34:2463–8.

23. Sarzi-Puttini P, Giorgi V, Sirotti S, Marotto D, Ardizzone S, Rizzardini G, Antinori S, Galli M. COVID-19, cytokines and immunosuppression: what can we learn from severe acute respiratory syndrome? Clin Exp Rheumatol. 2020;38:337–42.

24. Bhatia R, Sylaja PN, Srivastava MVP, et al. Consensus statement - suggested recommendations for acute stroke management during the COVID-19 pandemic: expert group on behalf of the Indian Stroke Association. Ann Indian Acad Neurol. 2020;23:S15–23.

25. Li Y, Li M, Wang M, Zhou Y, Chang J, Xian Y, Wang D, Mao L, Jin H, Hu B. Acute cerebrovascular disease following COVID-19: a single center, retrospective, observational study. Stroke Vasc Neurol. 2020;5:279.

26. Baracchini C, Pieroni A, Viaro F, Cianci V, Cattelan AM, Tiberio I, Munari M, Causin F. Acute stroke management pathway during Coronavirus-19 pandemic. Neurol Sci. 2020;41:1003–5.

27. Khosravani H, Rajendram P, Notario L, Chapman MG, Menon BK. Protected code stroke: hyperacute stroke management during the coronavirus disease 2019 (COVID-19) pandemic. Stroke. 2020;51:1891–5.

28. AHA/ASA Stroke Council Leadership. Temporary emergency guidance to US Stroke Centers during the coronavirus disease 2019 (COVID-19) pandemic. Stroke. 2020;51:1910–2.

29. Dogra S, Jain R, Cao M, et al. Hemorrhagic stroke and anticoagulation in COVID-19. J Stroke Cerebrovasc Dis. 2020;29:104984.

Posterior Reversible Encephalopathy Syndrome (PRES) and Meningo-Encephalitis in COVID

4

Ornella Manara, Giulio Pezzetti, and Simonetta Gerevini

Neurological symptoms described in COVID-19 infected patients can also occur in a more inflammatory related setting as in case of posterior reversible encephalopathy syndrome (PRES) that can be associated with SARS-CoV2 infection due to the massive cytokine storm, damage to endothelium and vasogenic oedema. At brain imaging, quite symmetric bilateral focal or confluent vasogenic oedema with posterior parietal and occipital lobe involvement are found. In severe cases like in COVID-setting, PRES can be complicated by ischemia or haemorrhage: we then describe in the atlas two cases of classic and complicated COVID-related PRES.

Another severe complication of SARS-CoV-2 infection can be meningo-encephalitis due to hypoxic/metabolic alterations in a virus-triggered inflammatory response setting. Altered consciousness, seizures, coma are key clinical features. Neuroimaging reveals cortical and subcortical T2/FLAIR signal alterations. Even if SARS-CoV2 is rarely detected in cerebrospinal fluid (CSF), in presence of suggestive clinical and imaging findings, especially if associated with anosmia or dysgeusia, diagnosis of COVID-related meningoencephalitis can be done, as extensively discussed in Chap. 2.

O. Manara · G. Pezzetti · S. Gerevini (✉)
Neuroradiology Department, Papa Giovanni XXIII Hospital, Bergamo, Italy
e-mail: omanara@asst-pg23.it; gpezzetti@asst-pg23.it; sgerevini@asst-pg23.it

4.1 Posterior Reversible Encephalopathy Syndrome (PRES) in COVID-19 Setting

Posterior reversible encephalopathy syndrome (PRES) is characterized by acute onset of severe headache (25–55% of cases), nausea and vomiting, alterations in consciousness, partial or generalized seizures, status epilepticus (75–85% of cases) and visual disturbances (20–40%) [1–4]. PRES happens more frequently in young to middle-aged people, with a women predominance. If promptly diagnosed and appropriately treated, PRES can be, completely reversible in days–weeks. However, there can be irreversible severe complications like brainstem involvement, ischemia and haemorrhagic transformation, responsible for long-term neurological deficits or even death.

PRES can be triggered by different clinical entities: the most common aetiologies are (pre)-eclampsia, infection, sepsis, shock, hypertension, autoimmune disease, immunosuppressive treatments [1–4].

The pathogenesis of PRES is not exactly known.

Three main pathogenetic theories for PRES have been proposed, each of them has some limitations.

1. "Breakthrough theory": rapidly developing hypertension causes a breakdown in brain auto-

regulation leading to blood–brain barrier (BBB) collapse, hyper perfusion with protein and fluid extravasation and vasogenic oedema [5, 6].

2. "Vasospasm theory": PRES is caused by vasospasm with subsequent ischemia (overlap with Reversible cerebral vasoconstriction syndrome, RCVS) [5, 6].

3. "Toxic theory": PRES is triggered by endothelial damage caused by endogenous or exogenous toxins (preeclampsia, sepsis) [6, 7] via increased leukocyte trafficking, decreased production of endothelium-derived vasorelaxants and disproportioned release of proinflammatory and vasoconstrictive cytokines [8–13].

COVID-19 infection and PRES share multiple risk factors, responsible for loss of homeostatic regulation of blood flow to the brain, increased susceptibility to blood pressure changes and brain oedema [14, 15].

1. Renal failure is a strong predictor of the development of PRES (up to 55% of cases) [16]. The cytokine storm (fever, increased levels of ferritin, IL-6, TNF-α, LDH, CRP, D-dimer), typical of SARS-CoV2 infection, may be also responsible or associated with development of PRES, by means of blood–brain barrier (BBB) breakdown, increased vascular permeability and upregulation of vascular endothelial growth factor (VEGF) in hypoxic condition [14, 16].

2. Labile arterial blood pressure. Many cases of PRES in COVID-19 are seen in patients with relatively moderate blood pressure fluctuations as a possible consequence of SARS-CoV2-induced endothelial dysfunction.

3. Endothelial injury, key factor in PRES, is part of COVID-19 spectrum: SARS-CoV2, by means of the spike protein S1, binds to the angiotensin-converting enzyme 2 (ACE2) receptor leading to an increase in blood pressure and alteration of the endothelial layer [14, 17].

4. Hypoxia is a well-known trigger of inflammation at local and systemic levels [14, 18, 19].

5. Immunomodulatory-like and monoclonal drugs such as tocilizumab, known to induce PRES by means of endothelial modulation properties, are largely used in COVID-19 patients [20, 21].

PRES-associated haemorrhages, more frequent in COVID-19 setting, can be explained by coagulopathy, often in terms of disseminated intravascular coagulation syndrome with liver dysfunction and consumption of clotting factors [14].

As pure clinical diagnosis of PRES can be challenging, imaging is mandatory also in a prognostic fashion.

4.1.1 Brain Imaging in COVID-Related PRES

In case of COVID-19 infection the imaging presentation of PRES doesn't differ from the typical one, but in the published cases seems to be more extensive.

At CT and MRI, PRES is characterized by a symmetric bilateral vasogenic oedema with classic posterior parietal and occipital lobe involvement [22] (the middle cerebral artery (MCA)–posterior cerebral artery (PCA) border zone). Calcarine and paramedian occipital lobe is usually spared. Subcortical white matter and cortical grey matter can be involved, depending upon the severity of the disease. CT is less sensitive than MRI in detecting the initial findings, with a normality rate of CT around 22% [2, 22, 23]. The most sensitive MRI sequence is Fluid Attenuated Inversion Recovery (FLAIR). Diffusion-weighted (DWI) is pivotal to distinguish classic and reversible PRES (vasogenic oedema, high signal on apparent diffusion coefficient–ADC–map) from complicated, irreversible cases (cytotoxic ischemic oedema, high signal on DWI, low signal on ADC map). Quantitative assessment of ADC maps can detect mild alterations [24]. DWI can be very useful in the prediction of irreversible tissue damage. Diffusion-tensor imaging (DTI) reveals anisotropy loss in posterior regions [24]. At magnetic resonance spectroscopy imaging (MRS) [25] there are slowly reversible metabolic abnormalities with increased choline and creatinine levels and mildly decreased *N*-acetyl aspartate in normal and abnormal appearing brain regions on conventional MRI sequences.

The main patterns of PRES include:

1. Parieto-occipital dominance (typical) [2, 23, 26].
2. Holo-hemispheric involvement at watershed zones (anterior cerebral artery [ACA]/MCA/ PCA border zones) [23, 26].
3. Superior frontal sulcus distribution (ACA/ MCA border zones): isolated involvement of mid and posterior aspect of superior frontal sulcus [2, 23, 26].
4. Central variant (<5% of cases) with involvement of temporal lobes, deep white matter, basal ganglia, brainstem, splenium of corpus callosum and cerebellum [26].
5. Overlapping or asymmetric expression of the previous-described patterns.

Imaging findings are usually reversible in days to weeks after treatment. In severe cases (around 15–20% of patients), PRES may progress to infarction (cytotoxic oedema with diffusion restriction, low ADC values) or haemorrhage, both petechial and intraparenchymal (hypointensity areas on Gradient Echo (GRE) T2* or Susceptibility-Weighted Imaging (SWI) sequences). Parenchymal or leptomeningeal contrast enhancement may be seen in subacute phase. If complicated or in cases of brainstem involvement, PRES tends to be irreversible with parenchymal damage resulting in encephalomalacia [2, 23, 26, 27].

In most patients with PRES (85%) there are overlapping features with RCVS (Reversible cerebral vasoconstriction syndrome) characterized by reversible focal vasoconstriction, vasodilatation and "string of bead" appearance of medium and small arteries, revealed by CT Angiogram (CTA) or catheter angiography [23, 28].

The main imaging differential diagnoses of PRES, based on the distribution of the lesions, are:

(a) Hypoxic ischemic encephalopathy: similar pattern of oedema. Involvement of the deep grey matter is peculiar in HIE [29].

(b) Bilateral subacute posterior border-zone infarcts: unilateral vascular distribution, cytotoxic oedema [29–31].
(c) Basilar top syndrome: involvement of medial occipital lobe and thalami.
(d) Vasculitis: reversibility of PRES lesions might be of help.
(e) Reversible brain oedema in post-ictal state and seizures: hippocampi and splenium of corpus callosum are usually involved [23].
(f) Encephalitis: involvement of grey and white matter.

4.1.2 Case Description

In this chapter, we extensively present clinical cases as we faced them: clinical setting first and images as last of this chapter.

4.1.2.1 Case 1

In April 2020, a previously healthy 56-year-old man presented with 10 days of dyspnoea, headache, fever, and cough. He tested positive for COVID-19 and was treated with hydrossicloroquine and steroids. Blood pressure range was 145–190/80–95 mmHg, with no metabolic derangements.

After days of hospitalization, due to persistence of altered mental status in spite of weaning sedation, brain CT scan revealed cortico-subcortical mild hypodensity with swelling involving right anterior-middle aspect of frontal lobe, right posterior parietal lobe and left temporo-occipital region. No haemorrhagic contamination was seen. No evidence of intracranial arterial malformations or venous sinus thrombosis was seen at CT arterial and venous angiogram (not shown).

A brain contrast-enhanced MRI done after days of hospitalization revealed cortico-subcortical predominant white matter T2 and FLAIR hyperintense signal alterations in right anterior-middle aspect of frontal lobe, right posterior parietal lobe, left temporo-occipital region and, in a lesser extent, left middle frontal area. There was hyperintensity on DWI (T2-shine through effect) with no diffusion restriction on ADC map and no haemorrhage in keeping with vasogenic oedema in a typical plus superior frontal sulcus pattern of PRES. No alterations were seen of magnetic resonance angiogram. After Gadolinium, there was mild punctate and linear enhancement in the previously described areas especially in right fronto-parietal regions, in keeping with BBB injury. On Day 20 since hospitalization, he had seizures with rightward gaze deviation and right arm and leg shaking. He was treated with levetiracetam and valproic acid. His mental status improved during the following weeks. Patient was discharged after 3 weeks of hospitalization in discrete clinical conditions (Figs. 4.1 and 4.2).

4.1.2.2 Case 2

At the beginning of March 2020, a 21-year-old young man affected by Alport syndrome (with mildly elevated creatinine levels) accessed to our emergency department referring 5 days of dyspnea, headache, fever, and dry cough. He tested positive for SARS-CoV2 virus on a nasopharyngeal swab. He was treated with hydrossicloroquine and steroids. His hospital course was complicated with mild respiratory failure requiring CPAP positioning. On hospital Day 15, an un-enhanced head MRI was obtained because of persistently poor mental status and revealed typical bilateral and quite symmetric cortical-subcortical T2-FLAIR signal hyperintensity with high signal in DWI and in ADC map in temporo-occipital regions and in posterior and mesial aspect of parietal lobe. Anterior and middle lateral aspects of frontal lobes, especially on the right-hand side, were also involved (superior frontal sulcus pattern). Punctate hyperintense lesions in right cerebellar hemisphere. No haemorrhagic components. These findings were in keeping with PRES alterations with typical posterior pattern associated with superior frontal sulcus involvement.

His mental status slowly improved. Patient was discharged after 4 weeks of hospitalization in good clinical conditions (Fig. 4.3).

4.1.3   Discussion

We described two cases of COVID-related PRES. First case showed a complicated PRES brain involvement with BBB damage expressed by punctate leptomeningeal and cortical contrast enhancement. The second one is a classic case of non-complicated PRES without cytotoxic oedema or haemorrhage. Anyway, in both cases there is a mixed pattern of PRES, with typical posterior regions involvement associated with superior frontal sulcus pattern.

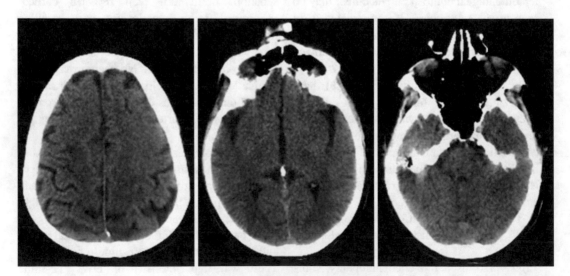

Fig. 4.1 Axial slices of brain non-contrast CT scan (16/04/20). Cortico-subcortical mild hypodensity with swelling involving right anterior-middle aspect of frontal lobe, right posterior parietal lobe and left temporo-occipital region

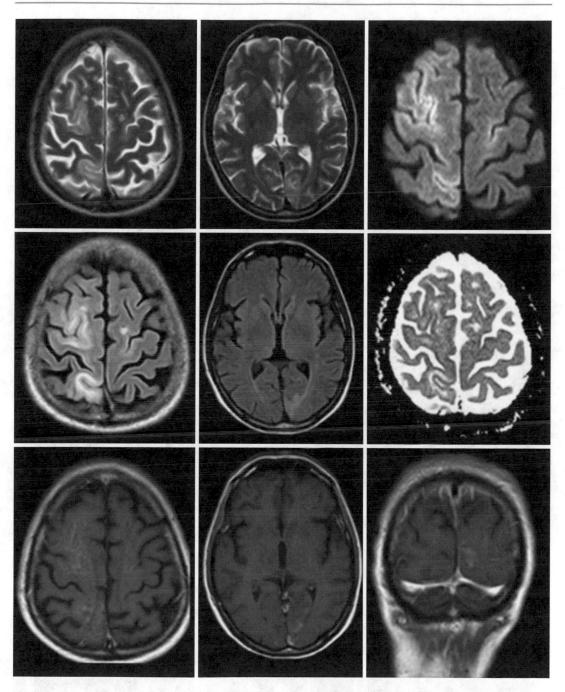

Fig. 4.2 Brain contrast-enhanced MRI scan (17/04/20). Cortico-subcortical T2-FLAIR hyperintense signal alterations in right anterior-middle aspect of frontal lobe, right posterior parietal lobe, left temporo-occipital region and, in a lesser extent, left middle frontal area. Hyperintensity on DWI (T2-shine through effect) with no diffusion restriction on ADC map and no haemorrhage (GRE sequence not shown). Mild punctate and linear enhancement especially in right fronto-parietal regions

From left to right and from upward to downward:

- *First row: axial T2-weighted sequences (two slices), axial diffusion-weighted imaging (DWI)*
- *Second row: axial fluid attenuated inversion recovery (FLAIR) sequences (two slices), axial apparent diffusion coefficient (ADC) map (ADC)*
- *Third row: axial post-Gadolinium T1-weighted sequences (two slices), coronal post-Gadolinium T1-weighted sequence*

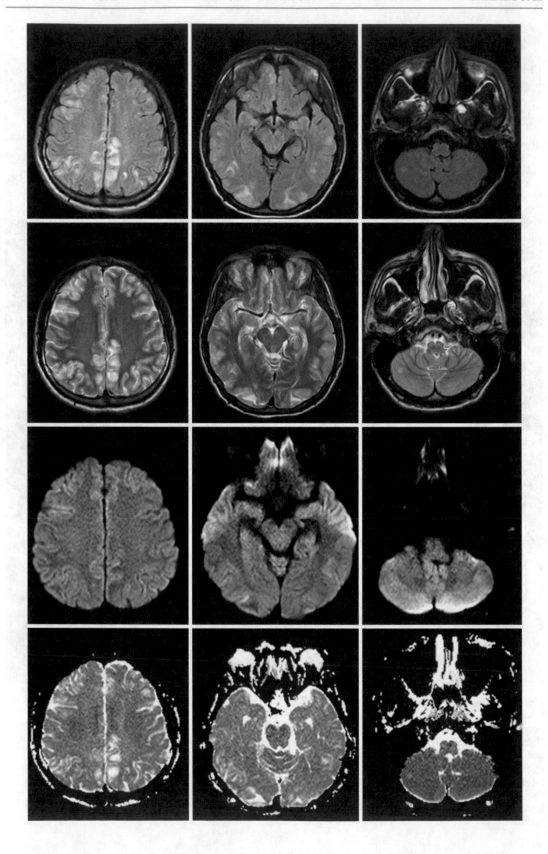

About 30 cases of PRES have been described since February 2020 in patients with positive SARS-CoV2 swab and congruous clinical and imaging pattern. To be mentioned is also a PRES case seen during postmortem imaging [32] in a COVID-19. According to the Literature, the majority of PRES patients had severe respiratory manifestations of COVID-19 requiring intensive respiratory support. PRES can develop also in asymptomatic COVID-19 patients [33]. The high number of COVID-19-related PRES cases can be also due to large use of interleukin 1 and 6 inhibitors (Anakinra and Tocilizumab) in COVID-19 therapy: these drugs can directly act on endothelial function favouriting typical PRES alterations [20, 34–37]. In 60% of patients with clinically suspected PRES brain MRI was normal. In about 40% of cases, typical PRES pattern is seen with often mild, posterior, bilateral, quite symmetric oedema [33]. In COVID-19 setting, as seen in our cases, there is an increased rate (10–30% of patients) of deep white matter, basal ganglia and cerebellum involvement as well as haemorrhagic contamination [14, 38, 39], cytotoxic oedema (diffusion restriction) and increased parenchymal and leptomeningeal contrast enhancement in a holo-hemispheric distribution with frequent basal ganglia and cerebellar involvement [14, 39].

Due to higher rate of complications, in all COVID-19 patients with suspected PRES it is pivotal to acquire GRE T2* or, better, SWI sequences (to reveal small and punctate haemorrhagic foci) and MRA in addition to the other morphologic sequences and DWI.

4.2   Meningo-Encephalitis in COVID-19 Setting

Viral meningoencephalitis is the result of human virus affecting brain and meninges and can involve any age group [40]. The prodrome of encephalitis is often nonspecific; the patients show neurologic manifestation such as fever, headache, nausea and vomiting, seizures and unconsciousness, altered sensorium, neurological deficit and coma. Many encephalitis cases have high morbidity and mortality.

With encephalopathy we mean a diffuse brain dysfunction of toxic, metabolic, hypoxic-ischemic, septic, inflammatory or immune-mediated aetiology. Primary encephalitis is due to direct involvement of CNS, while in secondary/post infectious encephalitis there is a CNS spreading of a viral infection located elsewhere in the body [40].

In viral encephalitis, some viruses are neurotropic (they specifically target the brain, spinal cord and/or peripheral nerves), others cause unselective collateral damage to CNS. The neurotropic viruses may reach the CNS by haematogenous, cerebrospinal fluid (CSF) or neural route e.g. Herpes Virus [41].

Brain damage in viral encephalitis results from the intracellular virus proliferation and from host inflammatory-immune response, against the virus or the infected cells.

The diagnosis is based on laboratory investigations on CSF analysis; neuroimaging has a critical and important role in early diagnosis and for follow-up [42].

Fig. 4.3 Brain MRI scan (24/03/20). Typical bilateral and quite symmetric cortical-subcortical T2-FLAIR signal hyperintensity with high signal in DWI and in ADC map in temporo-occipital regions and in posterior and mesial aspect of parietal lobe. Anterior and middle lateral aspects of frontal lobes, especially on the right-hand side, were also involved (superior frontal sulcus pattern). Punctate hyperintense lesions in right cerebellar hemisphere. No haemorrhagic components

From upward to downward:

- *First row: axial fluid attenuated inversion recovery (FLAIR) sequences (three slices)*
- *Second row: axial T2-weighted sequences (three slices)*
- *Third row: axial diffusion-weighted imaging (DWI) (three slices)*
- *Fourth row: axial apparent diffusion coefficient (ADC) map (ADC) (three slices)*

Magnetic resonance (MR) might reveal non-specific findings as vasogenic brain oedema and local or diffuse swelling, haemorrhages, necrosis and different patterns of enhancement, i.e. parenchymal and/or leptomeningeal [40, 43].

At macroscopic pathologic analysis, there are reduced transparency of the meninges, vascular congestion and local or diffuse swelling; microscopically infiltration by inflammatory cells is found [42].

Around 15 viral families (about 100 viruses) plus a non-viral agent (prion) may infect CNS [43, 44].

Certain viruses have a particular affinity for specific CNS cells (meningeal cells, oligodendrocytes, astrocytes and neurons) due to their cell-surface properties: based on the location of the signal abnormality, specific MRI diagnosis can be achieved [40, 42].

Herpes viruses replicate in neuronal and glial cells of the limbic system [41]; JC virus mainly involves oligodendrocytes in the thalamus, basal ganglia, cerebral cortex [45, 46]; Coxsachie involve the midbrain [47], Echo viruses, meningeal and ependymal cells [47].

Clinical presentation varies from asymptomatic to rapidly progressive and severe also with fatal outcome. Often, the severity of disease is not related to the virus itself but to the host inflammatory-immune systemic response the viral agent can trigger [40, 42].

The most common and early neurological manifestations in COVID-19 are myalgias, headache, dizziness, anosmia and dysgeusia. More severe symptoms of COVID-19 associated encephalitis/encephalopathy are fever, headache, seizure, focal neurological deficits, delirium, altered consciousness and coma [48, 49].

According to a retrospective review of 841 hospitalized patients with COVID-19 (mean age: 66.4 years), 57% had a neurological symptom [49, 50]. Altered consciousness (about 20% patients) usually occurs in old patients with severe disease [51]. Generalized myoclonus, aggravated by auditory and tactile stimuli, was described in severe cases of COVID-19-related CNS involvement: a post-infectious autoimmune pathogenesis was suspected [52].

MRI features of SARS-CoV-2-associated meningoencephalitis are nonspecific, congruous with a diffuse brain inflammatory condition: poorly delineated focal or diffuse T2/FLAIR hyperintensity of superficial and deep grey matter and/or white matter, basal ganglia/thalamus, areas of oedema, diffusion restriction, patchy haemorrhage, necrosis and variable enhancement can be found [53].

In COVID-19 associated encephalitis, CSF examination may show inflammatory changes (increased protein and/or cells). The presence of the virus SARS-CoV-2 within the CNS is related to neuro-invasiveness/neuro-tropism (the virus capacity to reach the CNS) and neurovirulence (the virus capacity to actively proliferate within the CNS). SARS-CoV-2 can enter the CNS via hematogenous dissemination or via retrograde pathway along olfactory nerves [54–56].

As other genetically similar neurotropic coronaviruses (HCoVs, SARS-CoV16, SARS-CoV27, SARS-CoV1), but with higher affinity, SARS-CoV2 enters a neural cell using the cell membrane-bound human angiotensin-converting enzyme 2 (ACE) receptor, widely expressed in the glial cells and in the brain stem nuclei with cardiorespiratory regulating effects [57, 58]. After ACE receptor binding, a cytokine storm is triggered with an important inflammatory response, blood–brain barrier breakdown [59] and increased destructive effects on CNS. Another possible pathogenetic mechanism involves a secondary hemophagocytic lymphohistiocytosis (sHLH) development resulting in a hyperinflammatory syndrome with fulminant hypercytokinemia responsible for fatal sepsis and multiorgan failure [60–62].

Plasmaferesis or hyperimmune plasma injection has been used as a treatment, with significative results [63, 64].

4.2.1 Case Description

4.2.1.1 Case 1

A 76-years-old male, with a previous history of arterial hypertension, atrial fibrillation in therapy, peripheral vascular disease, was taken to the

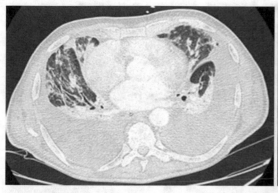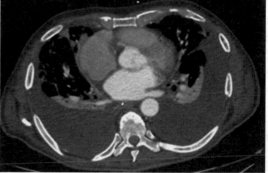

Fig. 4.4 Axial slices of chest CT (05/04/20) with lung (on the left) and mediastinum windows (on the right). Diffuse lung peri bronchial consolidations and ground glass alterations (interstitial pneumonia), associated with significant bilateral pleural effusion. No pulmonary thromboembolism

emergency department due to fever, dyspnoea, severe respiratory failure, altered mental status and coma. He was intubated the next day. During hospitalization he developed kidney failure requiring dialysis, important anaemia with need for blood transfusions, peripheral motor sensory polyneuropathy, episodes of atrial flutter. His clinical conditions were complicated with a septic shock, requiring vasopressor and multiple antibiotics. Chest CT scan revealed diffuse interstitial pneumonia; COVID-19 swab was positive. First brain CT was normal. At neurological examination he had discreet plastic hypertonus, with hints of asterixis. On a follow-up CT scan showing a diffuse hypodense alteration affecting the bi-hemispheric subcortical white matter, especially at the level of the semi-oval centres with associated multiple hypodense cortical-subcortical alterations. Brain MRI (see below) scan revealed diffuse signal alteration in keeping with encephalitic picture; the involvement of both thalami and the presence of both hemosiderin deposits and focal areas of diffusion restriction is consistent with acute necrotizing encephalopathy. At cerebrospinal fluid assessment with chemical-physical and cytological examination there were five nucleated elements, proteins >125, glucose value of 64. CFS PCR resulted positive for SARS-CoV-2. Under the suspicion of post viral autoimmune encephalitis, he underwent IV immunoglobulin G therapy for four cycles at a dose of 0.4 g/kg for 5 days, with progressive slow improvement of clinical conditions. He was dismissed from the hospital after about 3 months of hospitalization with a final diagnosis of SARS-CoV-2 related necrotizing encephalitis (Figs. 4.4, 4.5, 4.6, and 4.7).

4.2.1.2 Case 2

A 56-year-old man, with a previous history of arterial hypertension was taken to the emergency department due to dyspnoea, severe respiratory failure, altered mental status, increasing seizures and coma. He was immediately intubated. He developed septic shock, requiring vasopressor and various lines of antibiotics. Chest CT scan (not shown) revealed interstitial pneumonia; COVID-19 swab was positive.

At neurological examination he had plastic hypertonus. Urgent brain MRI (10/04/20) showed marked and diffuse T2-FLAIR hyperintensities with significant swelling involving the grey and white matter of bilateral fronto-parietal, temporo-occipital, temporo-polar regions and left posterior cingulum with striking left prevalence. Moreover, right thalamus, left thalamus and internal capsule, splenium of the corpus callosum (with left prevalence), left cerebellar hemisphere and vermis are affected. In all described regions there is diffusion alteration with significant restriction, hypointense on ADC map, especially in the right portion of the splenium, left cingulum and temporo-occipital lobe, consistent with mixed vasogenic and cytotoxic oedema.

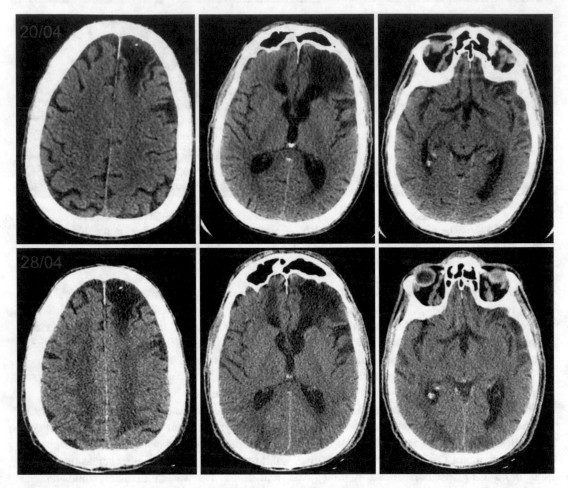

Fig. 4.5 Axial slices of Brain CT (20/04–28/04/20). In the first exam (upper row) no actual pathologic findings; post-traumatic porencephalic left frontal area. Follow-up exam (lower row) shows diffuse infra and supratentorial white matter hypodense alteration with sparing of U-fibres and cortical layer

Fig. 4.6 Brain contrast-enhanced MRI scan (29/04/20). Diffuse quite symmetric T2-FLAIR hyperintensity involving infra and supratentorial white matter with a predominant periventricular distribution with increased diffusion; corpus callosum and bilateral thalamic involvement (>right); punctate haemorrhagic foci are seen in right temporo-occipital region, thalami (>left) and cerebellar hemispheres. Small right parietal ischemic lesions. No significant contrast enhancement after Gadolinium injection. No vascular malformations

From upward to downward:

- *First row: axial T2-weighted sequences (three slices); axial fluid attenuated inversion recovery (FLAIR) sequences (three slices)*
- *Second row: axial T2-weighted sequences (three slices)*
- *Third row: axial diffusion-weighted imaging (DWI) (three slices)*
- *Fourth row: axial apparent diffusion coefficient (ADC) map (ADC) (three slices)*

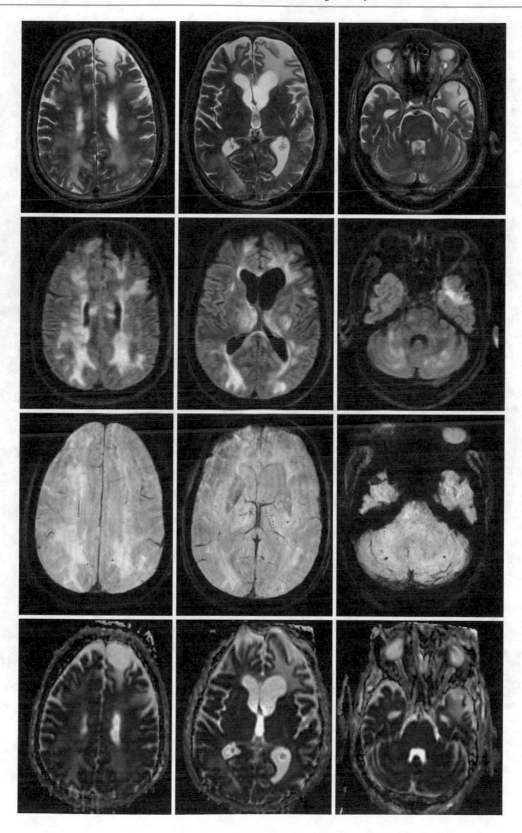

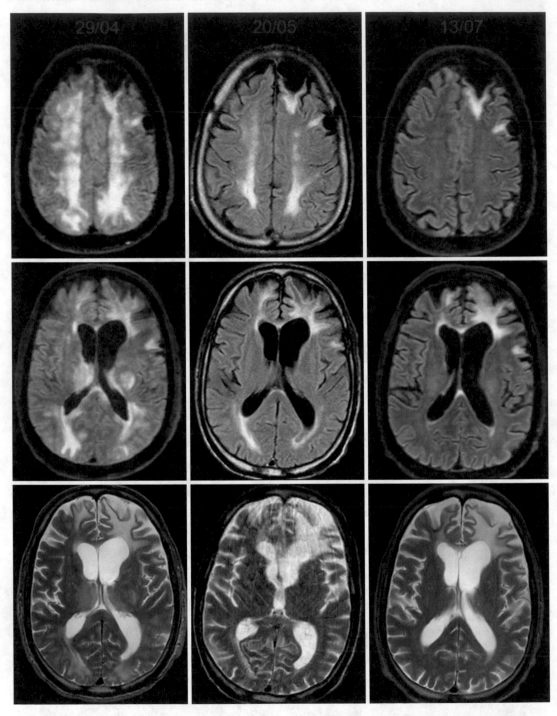

Fig. 4.7 Disease follow-up with brain contrast-enhanced MRI scans (29/04–20/05–13/07/20). Progressive improvement of brain white matter alterations. Minimal residual atrophy

From upward to downward:

- *First and second rows: axial fluid attenuated inversion recovery (FLAIR) sequences (different levels)*
- *Third row: axial T2-weighted sequences (three slices)*

Haemorrhagic methaemoglobin-hemosiderin contamination (mildly hyperintense on T1 and hypointense on T2-GRE T2*) was found in left temporo-occipital and cerebellar areas. Cortical laminar necrosis and faint contrast enhancement in keeping with altered BBB can be also appreciated. There was significant mass effect with right-sided midline shift, trans-falcine cingular gyrus herniation, right displacement of fourth ventricle and brain stem and downward position of cerebellar tonsils. Imaging findings were in keeping with severe acute haemorrhagic encephalitic pattern.

On brain CT scan performed after 10 days due to clinical worsening with ataxia and cerebellar signs, there was a huge oedematous left cerebellar parenchymal hematoma (about 45 × 30 mm) with signs of different age bleeding. Diffuse cortico-subcortical hypodensity and punctate haemorrhagic lesions were also seen.

Follow-up brain MRI performed after 15 days, in the previously involved brain areas there was diffuse cortico-subcortical atrophy with malacic alterations and diffuse cortical laminar necrosis (T1 cortical hyperintensity) and BBB residual breakdown with faint contrast enhancement. Normal evolution of the left hemispheric cerebellar hematoma. Oedema and mass effect are quite completely resolved with e-vacuo enlargement of the lateral ventricles.

At cerebrospinal fluid assessment with chemical-physical and cytological examination there were some nucleated cells, proteins >150, glucose value of 72. CSF PCR tested positive for SARS-CoV2. He underwent IV immunoglobulin G therapy for three cycles at a dose of 0.4 g/kg for 5 days, with slow improvement of clinical conditions (Figs. 4.8, 4.9, 4.10, and 4.11).

4.2.1.3 Case 3

A 56-year-old male, HCV positive. In March 2020, he was taken to emergency department after being found in coma but spontaneously breathing. He was intubated at home. First two nasopharyngeal SARS-CoV-2 swabs were negative. He was admitted to Intensive Care Unit.

Brain CT and EEG were negative; chest CT revealed compact parenchymal consolidation with air bronchogram and scissure delimitation in the basal-posterior and superior segments of the inferior lobes. On the right, consolidation involved also the anterior, posterior and apical portions of the upper lobe. Diffuse peribroncovascular infiltrates with predominantly ground glass patterns are associated, with relative sparing of the lower parts of the middle lobe and lingula.

Due to massive increase of inflammatory indices (PCT 158, PCR 45), he was treated with Piperacillin/Tazobactam + Metronidazole then replaced with Amoxicillin/Clavulanate + Clarithromycin, with slow improvement of clinical picture.

Then, hospitalization complicated with sepsis and Crush syndrome with renal insufficiency (and hepatic insufficiency). He remained in a state of coma (opening eyes to painful stimulus, hint of flexion). Due to persistent severe respiratory failure, repeated BAL tested positive for SARS-CoV-2 (on 24/3/2020). Subsequent BAL of 18/4 and 23/4 were negative.

Brain CT revealed diffuse supratentorial periventricular and corona radiata white matter hypodensities with no haemorrhagic components.

During hospitalization in infectious diseases unit he was put on CPAP. He was then transferred in intensive care unit and intubated again due to infection and septic shock. Blood cultures were positive for Enterococcus faecium treated with Linezolid with benefit (suspended on 20/4).

Brain MRI with MR angiography revealed supratentorial white matter, especially in bilateral frontal and parietal regions, with sparing of the U-shaped fibres, showed altered T2-FLAIR hyperintense signal with increased diffusion. On SWI sequence there were multiple deposits of haemoglobin degradation products in the posterior fossa and in the supratentorial compartment both in brain tissue (including the corpus callosum) and in the subarachnoid spaces. Gliotic-malacic ischemic stabilized ischemia in the right pallidum. Compared to the previous CT scan there was a progressive enlargement of the supratentorial ventricles. No areas of contrast enhancement. There was marked hypotrophy of olfactory bulbs with left prevalence.

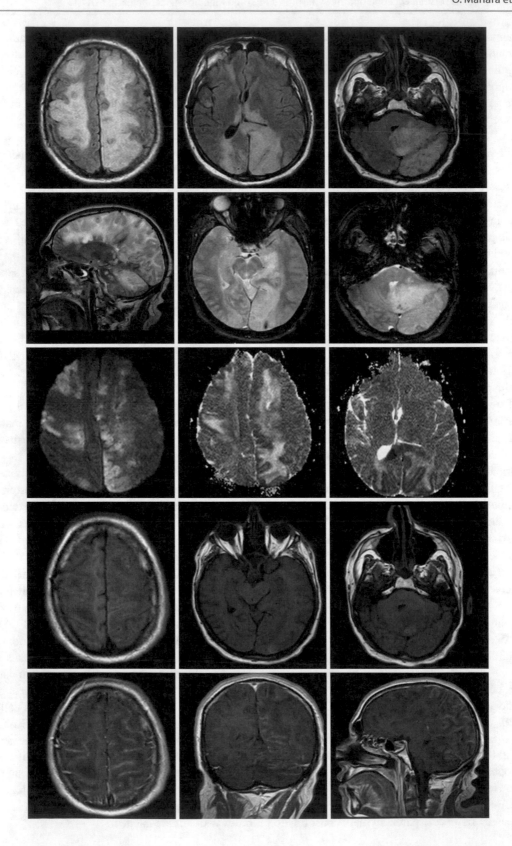

The findings were in keeping with COVID-related encephalopathy with marked atrophy: no specific therapies were done (Figs. 4.12, 4.13, 4.14, and 4.15).

4.2.1.4 Case 4

A 56-year-old male, with previous history of arterial hypertension in therapy with olmesartan 20 mg/day, chronic cerebral vasculopathy and mild cognitive impairment, on 1/5/20 was found unconscious on the ground at home feverish with sphincter release. He was taken to our emergency department where he performed un-enhanced brain CT revealing bilateral subarachnoid haemorrhage, especially in the cingular region (>left). Moreover, there are some hypodense periventricular (>posterior) white matter alterations, in keeping with chronic cerebral vasculopathy and bilateral capsulo-lenticular stabilized ischemic lesions. Mild enlargement of the ventricular system. Subsequent CT angiogram (not shown) was normal.

Chest X-ray showed diffuse confluent interstitial-alveolar alterations in both lungs with relative sparing of the apical regions.

Antibiotic therapy with ceftriaxone and azithromycin (continued for 5 days) associated with methylprednisolone (1 mg/kg for 5 days then gradually decreasing) was started. He was intubated with good respiratory exchanges.

At blood tests: white cells 7380 (6320 neutrophils), Haemoglobin 15, platelets 134, AST 81, ALT 49, LDH 468; SARS CoV2 nasopharyngeal swab was positive. The patient was enrolled in the study protocol for Remdesivir drug, administered for 10 days. He also underwent hyperimmune plasma experimental treatment. In the following days there was a clinical worsening with progressive disorientation and expressive aphasia, after neurological consult, diagnostic lumbar puncture was performed: at CSF exam there were 2000 red cells, glycorrhachia and protidorrachia were normal. PCRs for herpes viruses, enteroviruses and SARS-Cov2 were negative. EEG showed globally slowed activity.

Brain MRI with MRA (08/05/20) revealed diffuse confluent supratentorial periventricular and deep white matter T2-FLAIR high signal intensity alteration with increased diffusion and mild increased perfusion. Left callosal area of contrast enhancement and haemorrhagic contamination. Diffuse punctate infra and supratentorial white matter micro haemorrhagic–microthrombotic lesions. Small acute ischemic lesions in the posterior middle third of the left corona radiata. Olfactory bulbs were hypotrophic with left prevalence. In view of SARS-CoV-2 infection and rapid evolution of the clinical picture, findings were in keeping with haemorrhagic COVID-related encephalitis.

At follow-up brain MRI scan performed on 20/05/20 there was minimal reduction in left callosal contrast-enhanced alteration. Other findings were stable.

Fig. 4.8 Brain contrast-enhanced MRI scan (10/04/20). Marked and diffuse T2-FLAIR hyperintensities with tissue swelling involving the grey and white matter of bilateral fronto-parietal, temporo-occipital, temporo-polar regions and left posterior cingulum with left prevalence. Right thalamus, left thalamus and internal capsule, splenium of the corpus callosum (with left prevalence), left cerebellar hemisphere and vermis are affected. In all regions there is significant diffusion restriction especially in the right portion of the splenium. Haemorrhagic contamination in left temporo-occipital and cerebellar areas. Cortical laminar necrosis and faint contrast enhancement was seen. Significant mass effect with right-sided midline shift, trans-falcine cingular gyrus herniation, right displacement of fourth ventricle and brain stem and downward position of cerebellar tonsils

From left to right and from upward to downward:

- *First row: axial fluid attenuated inversion recovery (FLAIR) sequences (three slices)*
- *Second row: sagittal T2-weighted sequence, axial Gradient Echo T2* sequence (two slices)*
- *Third row: axial diffusion-weighted imaging (DWI, one slice) and apparent diffusion coefficient (ADC) map (two slices)*
- *Fourth row: axial T1-weighted sequences (three slices)*
- *Fifth row: axial, coronal and sagittal post-Gad T1-weighted sequence*

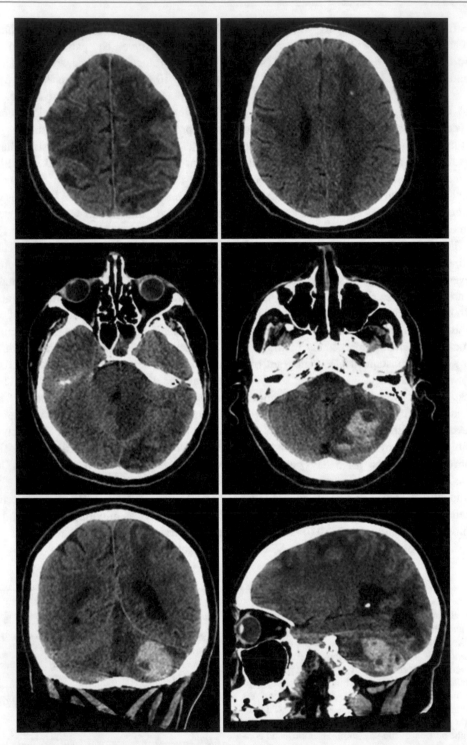

Fig. 4.9 Brain multiplanar non-contrast CT scan (19/04/20). Huge oedematous left cerebellar parenchymal hematoma (about 45 × 30 mm) with signs of different age bleeding. Diffuse cortico-subcortical hypodensity was seen in the MRI signal alteration areas. Punctate haemorrhagic lesions were seen also in left posterior temporo-occipital and superior frontal lobe

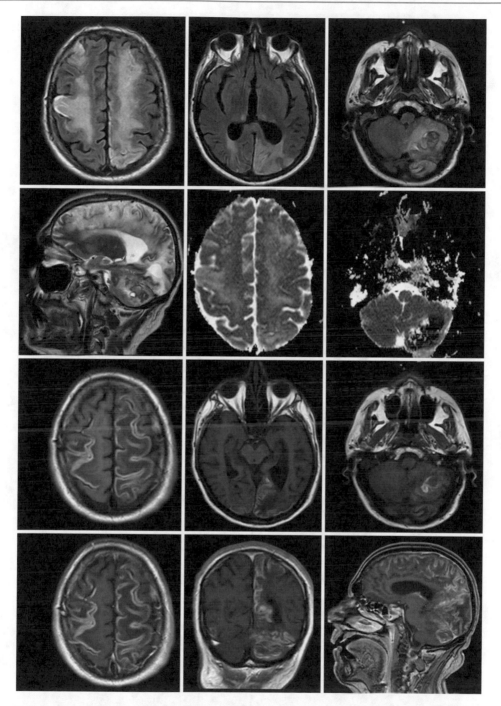

Fig. 4.10 Brain contrast-enhanced MRI scan (24/04/20). In the previously involved brain areas, there was diffuse cortico-subcortical atrophy with malacic alterations and diffuse cortical laminar necrosis and BBB residual breakdown with faint contrast enhancement. Normal evolution of the left hemispheric cerebellar haematoma. Quite complete resolution of oedema and mass effect with e-vacuo enlargement of the lateral ventricles

From left to right and from upward to downward:

- *First row: axial fluid attenuated inversion recovery (FLAIR) sequences (three slices)*
- *Second row: sagittal T2-weighted sequence, axial diffusion-weighted imaging (DWI, one slice) and apparent diffusion coefficient (ADC) map (one slice)*
- *Third row: axial T1-weighted sequences (three slices)*
- *Fourth row: axial, coronal and sagittal post-Gad T1-weighted sequence*

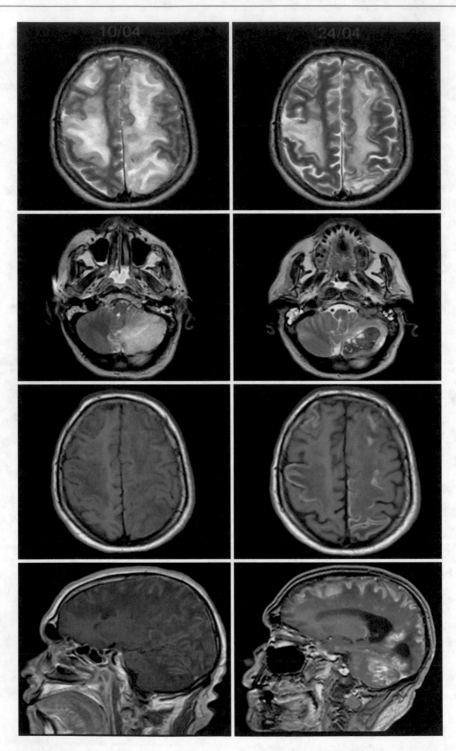

Fig. 4.11 Comparison between MRI scan of 10/04 (left) and 24/04/20 (right)

From upward to downward:
- *First and second rows: axial T2-weighted sequences*
- *Third row: axial T1-weighted sequences (three slices)*
- *Fourth row: sagittal post-Gad T1-weighted sequence*

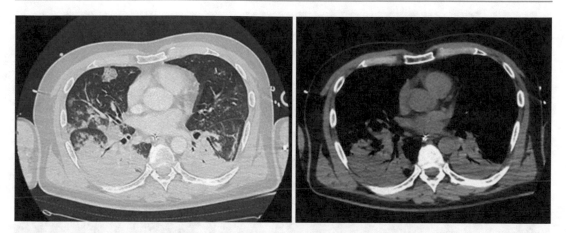

Fig. 4.12 Axial slices of chest CT (07/03/20) with lung (on the left) and mediastinum windows (on the right). Bilateral basal consolidations and ground glass alterations

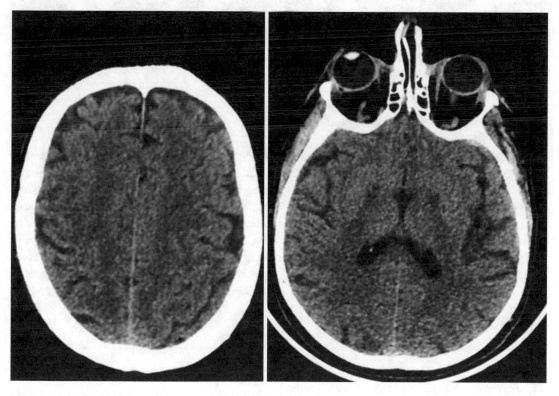

Fig. 4.13 Axial slices of brain CT (07/03/20). Normal findings

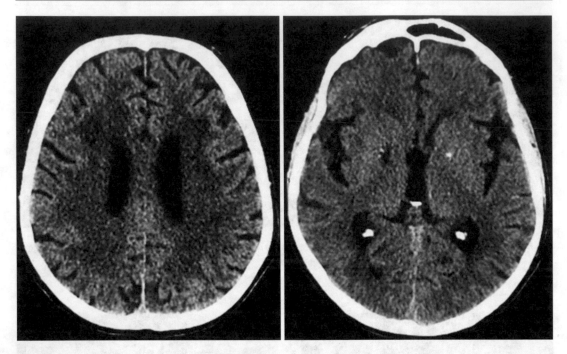

Fig. 4.14 Axial brain non-contrast CT scan (15/04/20). Diffuse supratentorial periventricular and corona radiata white matter hypodensity with no haemorrhagic components

The patient underwent a new diagnostic lumbar puncture on 25/05, always negative for SARS-CoV-2. His clinical conditions slowly improved: the patient was discharged after about 2 months of hospitalization.

In view of the clinical course, imaging findings and lab test a diagnosis of SARS-CoV-2-related encephalopathy/endothelitis was done. Due to the negativity of CSF viral test, a postviral immune-mediate mechanism was supposed (Figs. 4.16, 4.17, 4.18, and 4.19).

4.2.2 Discussion

Moriguchi et al. [55] and Zambreanu et al. [65] described cases of COVID-19-related meningo-encephalitis with involvement of limbic system and ventriculitis. SARS-CoV-2 RNA was not detected in the nasopharyngeal swab but in CSF.

Considering that in COVID associated encephalopathy brain imaging can also be completely normal [66–69], in many cases there is confluent and symmetric cytotoxic oedema (dif-

Fig. 4.15 Brain MRI scan (10/06/20). Diffuse confluent supratentorial periventricular white matter T2-FLAIR hyperintensities with increased diffusion. Right internal capsule involvement. Diffuse punctate micro haemorrhagic/micro thrombotic foci in supratentorial white matter, cerebellar hemispheres and corpus callosum as well as subarachnoid hemosiderin haemorrhagic components. No contrast enhancement (not shown). Marked olfactory bulbs hypotrophy with left prevalence

From left to right and from upward to downward:

- *First row: axial (two slices) and coronal (on olfactory bulbs) T2-weighted sequences*
- *Second row: axial, sagittal and coronal 3D fluid attenuated inversion recovery (FLAIR) reformatted sequences*
- *Third row: axial diffusion-weighted imaging (DWI, one slice), apparent diffusion coefficient (ADC) map (one slice) and T1-weighted sequences (one slice)*
- *Fourth row: axial Minimum intensity projection (MinIP) Susceptibility-weighted imaging (SWI)*

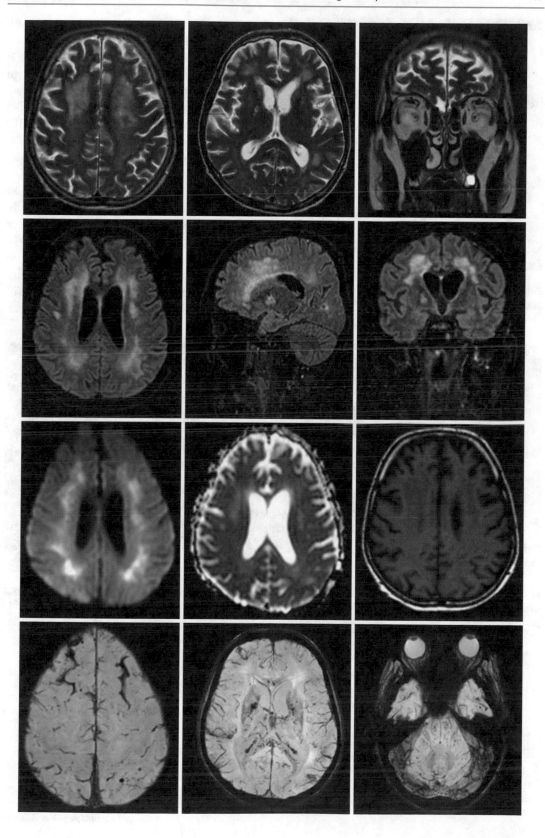

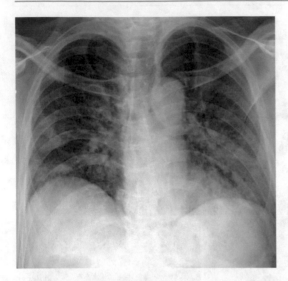

Fig. 4.16 Chest X-ray (01/05/20): diffuse confluent interstitial-alveolar alterations in both lungs with relative sparing of the apical regions

fusion restriction) in brain white matter, with sparing of subcortical U-fibres, similar to post-hypoxic leukoencephalopathy or high-altitude cerebral oedema. Leptomeningeal enhancement can be seen on post-contrast T1-weighted and fluid attenuated inversion recovery (FLAIR) sequences. Periventricular white matter T2/FLAIR hyperintensity and microbleeds can be associated in COVID-related microangiopathy setting [69].

COVID-19 is associated in about 5–25% of cases with hypoxia, silent or overt, especially in hospitalized intubated patients [70]. Silent hypoxia can be difficult to assess in particular in asymptomatic patients. However, in a recent case series [70] only one patient had clinically significantly low oxygen saturation (90%) at the time of presentation, suggesting that encephalopathy can

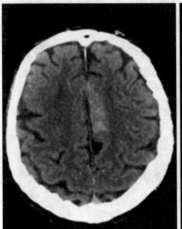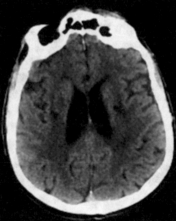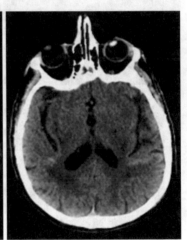

Fig. 4.17 Axial brain non-contrast CT scan (18/05/20). Bilateral subarachnoid haemorrhage, especially in the cingular region (>left). Moreover, there are some hypodense periventricular (>posterior) white matter alterations, in keeping with chronic cerebral vasculopathy and bilateral capsulo-lenticular stabilized ischemic lesions. Mild enlargement of the ventricular system

Fig. 4.18 Brain MRI scan (20/05/20). Diffuse confluent supratentorial periventricular and deep white matter T2-FLAIR high signal intensity alteration with increased diffusion and mild increased perfusion. Left callosal area of contrast enhancement and haemorrhagic contamination. Diffuse punctate infra and supratentorial white matter micro haemorrhagic–microthrombotic lesions. Olfactory bulbs hypotrophy with left prevalence

From left to right and from upward to downward:

- *First row: axial, sagittal and coronal 3D fluid attenuated inversion recovery (FLAIR) reformatted sequences*
- *Second row: axial (one slice) and coronal (on olfactory bulbs) T2-weighted sequence; dynamic susceptibility contrast (DSC) perfusion map (cerebral blood volume, rCBV)*
- *Third row: axial Minimum intensity projection (MinIP) Susceptibility-weighted imaging (SWI)*
- *Fourth row: axial, coronal and sagittal post-Gadolinium T1-weighted sequences*

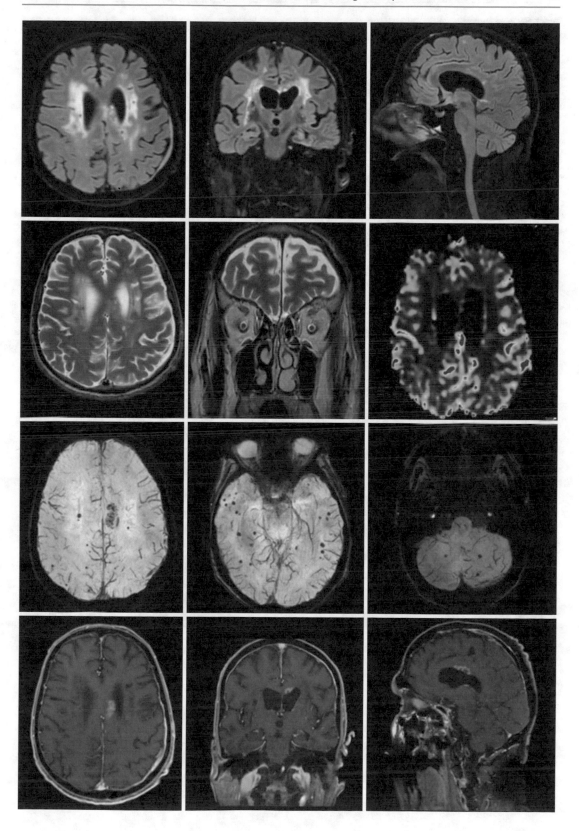

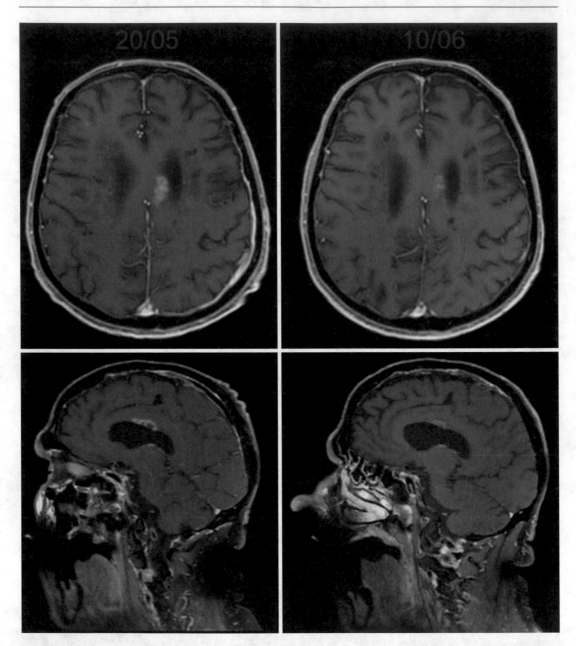

Fig. 4.19 Comparison between brain MRI scan of 20/05 and 10/06/20. Minimal reduction in left callosal contrast-enhanced alteration. The other findings are stable. *Axial* *(upper row) and sagittal (lower row) post-Gadolinium T1-weighted sequences are shown*

occur even before a proper hypoxic status. Grey matter, basal ganglia and brain stem can be involved as well as white matter, raising the suspicion for encephalitis even in the absence of other known causative factors.

So far, some peculiar COVID-19-related encephalitis patterns have been described:

1. COVID-19 can involve predominantly the white matter of brain, brainstem and spinal

cord with a suggested postviral demyelination mechanism, an immune-mediated inflammatory demyelinating disorder occurring within days to weeks after viral infection. In these cases, it is not the virus itself but the host-enhanced immune and inflammatory response which can damage both white and grey matter. Up to July 2020, 12 cases of possible immune-mediated encephalitis and postviral polyneuropathies have been described in COVID-19, with a mean age of patients around 40s [55, 70–73]. Clinical presentation ranged from neuropsychiatric symptoms and coma, to brainstem involvement (like Bickerstaff brainstem encephalitis), to cranial nerve palsies, to peripheral polyradiculitis like Guillain–Barré and Miller Fisher syndromes [71–74].

Severe and lethal cases of acute/fulminant acute haemorrhagic leukoencephalitis, ANE, or acute disseminated encephalomyelitis (ADEM) have been described so far [75]. Acute necrotizing encephalopathy (ANE), probably related to severe cytokine storm, is characterized by symmetrical, multiple T2-FLAIR hyperintense lesions in the thalamus, basal ganglia, deep white matter and brainstem with scattered haemorrhagic foci. Clinically, patient presents with seizures, focal neurological deficit and coma. In acute disseminated encephalomyelitis (ADEM) white matter, brainstem, optic nerves and spinal cord are variably affected [76].

In some cases, CSF pleocytosis and anti-GD1b IgG and anti-Caspr2 antibodies were found, which correlated with more severe disease and poor outcome [77, 78]. No evidence of direct SARS-CoV2 CNS infection was found.
2. Mild encephalitis/encephalopathy with a reversible splenial lesion, already described in case of MERS [79].
3. COVID-19-associated meningoencephalitis with intracerebral haemorrhage and subdural hematoma [62].
4. Steroid-responsive encephalitis with normal brain imaging suggesting a hyperinflammatory mechanism [74].

5. COVID-related rhombencephalitis usually in a context of a wider systemic inflammatory process. This particular form of encephalitis with brainstem involvement has been associated so far with multiple sclerosis, Bechet disease, listeria monocytogenes infection, paraneoplastic syndrome, Epstein–Barr virus and tuberculosis [80]. Many cases remained of unknown origin.

In COVID-19-related encephalitis, it is challenging to demonstrate direct infection of neurons/glial cells by SARS-CoV-2 viral particles, as most of RT-PCR analyses from CSF were normal or nonspecific [81]. Only in few patients with encephalitic features test was positive [55, 82]. Anyway, in presence of clinical and MRI suggestive findings in a COVID-19 positive patient, especially if associated with anosmia or dysgeusia, a negative CSF viral test does not rule out the diagnosis of meningoencephalitis.

Acknowledgements Cases 1 and 2 of Sect. 4.1 and Case 2 of Sect. 4.2 courtesy of:

- E. D'Adda, MD; M.E. Fruguglietti, MD; Neurologist Stroke Unit Cerebrovascular Dept; ASST Crema Hospital
- M. Borghetti MD, G. Benelli MD; Radiology Unit, Cerebrovascular Dept; ASST Crema Hospital
- G. Merli MD, G. Lupi MD, Department of Anesthesia and Critical Care Medicine, ASST Crema Hospital

References

1. Hinchey J, Chaves C, Appignani B, et al. A reversible posterior leukoencephalopathy syndrome. N Engl J Med. 1996;334(8):494–500. https://doi.org/10.1056/NEJM199602223340803.
2. Bartynski WS. Posterior reversible encephalopathy syndrome, part 1 and 2: fundamental imaging and clinical features. AJNR Am J Neuroradiol. 2008;29:1036–42. https://doi.org/10.3174/ajnr.A0928.
3. Bakshi R, Bates VE, Mechtler LL, et al. Occipital lobe seizures as the major clinical manifestation of reversible posterior leukoencephalopathy syndrome: magnetic resonance imaging findings. Epilepsia. 1998;39(3):295–9. https://doi.org/10.1111/j.1528-1157.1998.tb01376.x.

4. Fugate JE, Claassen DO, Cloft HJ, et al. Posterior reversible encephalopathy syndrome: associated clinical and radiologic findings. Mayo Clin Proc. 2010;85(5):427–32. https://doi.org/10.4065/mcp.2009.0590.

5. Miller TR, Shivashankar R, Mossa-Basha M, et al. Reversible cerebral vasoconstriction syndrome, part 1: epidemiology, pathogenesis, and clinical course. AJNR Am J Neuroradiol. 2015;36:1392–9. https://doi.org/10.3174/ajnr.A4214.

6. Schwartz RB, Jones KM, Kalina P, et al. Hypertensive encephalopathy: findings on CT, MR imaging, and SPECT imaging in 14 cases. AJR Am J Roentgenol. 1992;159:379–83. https://doi.org/10.2214/ajr.159.2.1632361.

7. Calabrese LH, Dodick DW, Schwedt TJ, et al. Narrative review: reversible cerebral vasoconstriction syndromes. Ann Intern Med. 2007;146:34–44. https://doi.org/10.7326/0003-4819-146-1-200701020-00007.

8. Chen SP, Fuh JL, Wang SJ, et al. Magnetic resonance angiography in reversible cerebral vasoconstriction syndromes. Ann Neurol. 2010;67:648–56. https://doi.org/10.1002/ana.21951.

9. Aird WC. The role of the endothelium in severe sepsis and multiple organ dysfunction syndrome. Blood. 2003;101:3765–77. https://doi.org/10.1182/blood-2002-06-1887.

10. Bartynski WS, Tan HP, Boardman JF, et al. Posterior reversible encephalopathy syndrome after solid organ transplantation. AJNR Am J Neuroradiol. 2008;29:924–30. https://doi.org/10.3174/ajnr.A0960.

11. Gupta S, Kaplan MJ. Pathogenesis of systemic lupus erythematosus. Rheumatology. 7th ed. Philadelphia, PA: Elsevier; 2019. p. 1154–9.

12. Loscalzo J. Endothelial injury, vasoconstriction, and its prevention. Tex Heart Inst J. 1995;22:180–4.

13. Sandoo A, van Zanten JJ, Metsios GS, et al. The endothelium and its role in regulating vascular tone. Open Cardiovasc Med J. 2010;4:302–12. https://doi.org/10.2174/1874192401004010302.

14. Franceschi AM, Ahmed O, Giliberto L, et al. Hemorrhagic posterior reversible encephalopathy syndrome as a manifestation of COVID-19 infection. AJNR Am J Neuroradiol. 2020;41(7):1173–6. https://doi.org/10.3174/ajnr.A6595.

15. Hernández-Fernández F, Valencia HS, Barbella-Aponte RA, et al. Cerebrovascular disease in patients with COVID-19: neuroimaging, histological and clinical description. Brain. 2020;143:3089. https://doi.org/10.1093/brain/awaa239.

16. Filatov A, Sharma P, Hindi F, et al. Neurological complications of coronavirus (COVID-19): encephalopathy. Cureus. 2020;12:e7352. https://doi.org/10.7759/cureus.7352.

17. Mehta P, McAuley DF, Brown M, et al. COVID-19: consider cytokine storm syndromes and immunosuppression. Lancet. 2020;395:1033–4. https://doi.org/10.1016/S0140-6736(20)30628-0.

18. Eltzschig HK, Carmeliet P. Hypoxia and inflammation. N Engl J Med. 2011;364:656–65. https://doi.org/10.1056/NEJMra0910283.

19. Bartels K, Grenz A, Eltzschig HK. Hypoxia and inflammation are two sides of the same coin. Proc Natl Acad Sci U S A. 2013;110:18351–2. https://doi.org/10.1073/pnas.1318345110.

20. Rosa Junior M, Borges EI, Fonseca APA, et al. Posterior reversible encephalopathy syndrome during treatment with tocilizumab in juvenile idiopathic arthritis. Arq Neuropsiquiatr. 2018;76:720–1. https://doi.org/10.1590/0004-282X20180093.

21. Cross SN, Ratner E, Rutherford TJ, et al. Bevacizumab-mediated interference with VEGF signalling is sufficient to induce a preeclampsia-like syndrome in nonpregnant women. Rev Obstet Gynecol. 2012;5:2–8.

22. McKinney AM, Short J, Truwit CL, et al. Posterior reversible encephalopathy syndrome: incidence of atypical regions of involvement and imaging findings. AJR Am J Roentgenol. 2007;189:904–12. https://doi.org/10.2214/AJR.07.2024.

23. Levitt M, Zampolin R, Burns J, et al. Posterior reversible encephalopathy syndrome and reversible cerebral vasoconstriction syndrome. Distinct Clinical Entities with Overlapping Pathophysiology. Radiol Clin N Am. 2019;57:1133–46. https://doi.org/10.1016/j.rcl.2019.07.001.

24. Covarrubias DJ, Luetmer PH, Campeau NG. Posterior reversible encephalopathy syndrome: prognostic utility of quantitative diffusion-weighted MR images. AJNR Am J Neuroradiol. 2002;23:1038–4.

25. Eichler FS, Wang P, Wityk RJ, et al. Diffuse metabolic abnormalities in reversible posterior leukoencephalopathy syndrome. AJNR Am J Neuroradiol. 2002;23(5):833–7.

26. Hefzy HM, Bartynski WS, Boardman JF, et al. Hemorrhage in posterior reversible encephalopathy syndrome: imaging and clinical features. AJNR Am J Neuroradiol. 2009;30(7):1371–9. https://doi.org/10.3174/ajnr.A1588.

27. Cruz-Flores S, de Assis Aquino Gondim F, Leira EC. Brainstem involvement in hypertensive encephalopathy: clinical and radiological findings. Neurology. 2004;62(8):1417–9. https://doi.org/10.1212/01.wnl.0000120668.73677.5f.

28. Pilato F, Distefano M, Calandrelli R. Posterior reversible encephalopathy syndrome and reversible cerebral vasoconstriction syndrome: clinical and radiological considerations. Front Neurol. 2020;11:34. https://doi.org/10.3389/fneur.2020.00034.

29. Muttikkal TJ, Wintermark M. MRI patterns of global hypoxic-ischemic injury in adults. J Neuroradiol. 2013;40:164–71. https://doi.org/10.1016/j.neurad.2012.08.002.

30. Wijdicks EF, Campeau NG, Miller GM. MR imaging in comatose survivors of cardiac resus-

citation. AJNR Am J Neuroradiol. 2001;22: 1561–5.

31. Ho ML, Rojas R, Eisenberg RL. Cerebral edema. AJR Am J Roentgenol. 2012;199:W258–73. https://doi.org/10.2214/AJR.11.8081.

32. Coolen T, Lolli V, Sadeghi N, et al. Early postmortem brain MRI findings in COVID-19 non-survivors. Neurology. 2020;95(14):e2016–27. https://doi.org/10.1212/WNL.0000000000010116.

33. Anand P, Lau HV, Chung DY, et al. Posterior reversible encephalopathy syndrome in patients with coronavirus disease 2019: two cases and a review of the literature. J Stroke Cerebrovasc Dis. 2020;29(11): 105212.

34. Gaensbauer JT, Press CA, Hollister JR, et al. Procalcitonin: a marker of infection not subverted by treatment with interleukin-6 receptor inhibition. Pediatr Infect Dis J. 2013;32(9):1040. https://doi.org/10.1097/INF.0b013e318295a3d0.

35. Kotani K, Miyamoto M, Ando H. The effect of treatments for rheumatoid arthritis on endothelial dysfunction evaluated by flow-mediated vasodilation in patients with rheumatoid arthritis. Curr Vasc Pharmacol. 2016;15(1):10–8. https://doi.org/10.2174/1570161114666161013113457.

36. Vallejo S, Palacios E, Romacho T, et al. The interleukin-1 receptor antagonist anakinra improves endothelial dysfunction in streptozotocin-induced diabetic rats. Cardiovasc Diabetol. 2014;13:158. https://doi.org/10.1186/s12933-014-0158-z.

37. Ikonomidis I, Lekakis JP, Nikolaou M, et al. Inhibition of interleukin-1 by anakinra improves vascular and left ventricular function in patients with rheumatoid arthritis. Circulation. 2008;117(20):2662–9. https://doi.org/10.1161/CIRCULATIONAHA.107.731877.

38. Doo FX, Kassim G, Lefton DR, et al. Rare presentations of COVID-19: PRES-like leukoencephalopathy and carotid thrombosis. Clin Imaging. 2020;69:94–101. https://doi.org/10.1016/j.clinimag.2020.07.007.

39. Rogg J, Baker A, Tung G. Posterior reversible encephalopathy syndrome (PRES): another imaging manifestation of COVID-19. Interdiscip Neurosurg. 2020;22:100808. https://doi.org/10.1016/j.inat.2020.100808.

40. Jayaraman K, Rangasami R, Chandrasekharan A. Magnetic resonance imaging findings in viral encephalitis: a pictorial essay. J Neurosci Rural Pract. 2018;9(4):556–60. https://doi.org/10.4103/jnrp.jnrp_120_18.

41. Egdell R, Egdell D, Solomon T. Herpes simplex virus encephalitis. BMJ. 2012;344:e3630. https://doi.org/10.1136/bmj.e3630.

42. Steiner I, Budka H, Chaudhuri A, et al. Viral meningoencephalitis: a review of diagnostic methods and guidelines for management. Eur J Neurol. 2010;17(8):999–e57. https://doi.org/10.1111/j.1468-1331.2010.02970.x.

43. Gupta RK, Soni N, Kumar S, et al. Imaging of central nervous system viral diseases. J Magn Reson Imaging. 2012;35(3):477–91. https://doi.org/10.1002/jmri.22830.

44. Finkenstaedt M, Szudra A, Zerr I, et al. MR imaging of Creutzfeldt-Jakob disease. Radiology. 1996;199(3):793–8. https://doi.org/10.1148/radiology.199.3.8638007.

45. Becker JT, Maruca V, Kingsley LA, et al. Multicenter AIDS Cohort Study. Factors affecting brain structure in men with HIV disease in the post-HAART era. Neuroradiology. 2011;54(2):113–21. https://doi.org/10.1007/s00234-011-0854-.

46. Shah R, Bag AK, Chapman PR, et al. Imaging manifestations of progressive multifocal leukoencephalopathy. Clin Radiol. 2010;65(6):431–9. https://doi.org/10.1016/j.crad.2010.03.001.

47. Misra UK, Kalita J, Phadke RV, et al. Usefulness of various MRI sequences in the diagnosis of viral encephalitis. Acta Trop. 2010;116(3):206–11. https://doi.org/10.1016/j.actatropica.2010.08.007.

48. Molimard J, Baudou E, Mengelle C, et al. Coxsackie B3-induced rhombencephalitis. Arch Pediatr. 2019;26(4):247–8. https://doi.org/10.1016/j.arcped.2019.02.013.

49. Asadi-Pooya AA, Simani L. Central nervous system manifestations of COVID-19: a systematic review. J Neurol Sci. 2020;413:116832. https://doi.org/10.1016/j.jns.2020.116832.

50. Hernandez-Fernandez F, Valencia HS, Barbella-Aponte RA, et al. Cerebrovascular disease in patients with COVID-19: neuroimaging, histological and clinical description. Brain. 2020;143:3089. https://doi.org/10.1093/brain/awaa239.

51. Mahammedi A, Saba L, Vagal A, et al. Imaging in neurological disease of hospitalized COVID-19 patients: an Italian multicenter retrospective observational study. Radiology. 2020;297:E270. https://doi.org/10.1148/radiol.2020201933.

52. Merkler AE, Parikh NS, Mir S, et al. Risk of ischemic stroke in patients with coronavirus disease 2019 (COVID-19) vs patients with influenza. JAMA Neurol. 2020;77:1. https://doi.org/10.1001/jamaneurol.2020.2730.

53. Garg RK, Paliwal VK, Gupta A. Encephalopathy in patients with COVID-19: a review. J Med Virol. 2020:1–17. https://doi.org/10.1002/jmv.26207.

54. Baig AM, Khaleeq A, Ali U, et al. Evidence of the COVID-19 virus targeting the CNS: tissue distribution, host-virus interaction, and proposed neurotropic mechanisms. ACS Chem Neurosci. 2020;11(7):995–8. https://doi.org/10.1021/acschemneuro.0c00174.

55. Moriguchi T, Harii N, Goto J, et al. A first case of meningitis/encephalitis associated with SARS-Coronavirus-2. Int J Infect Dis. 2020;94:55–8. https://doi.org/10.1016/j.ijid.2020.03.062.

56. Russell B, Moss C, Rigg A, et al. Anosmia and ageusia are emerging as symptoms in patients with

COVID-19: what does the current evidence say? Ecancermedicalscience. 2020;14:ed98. https://doi.org/10.3332/ecancer.2020.ed98.

57. Hamming I, Timens W, Bulthuis M, et al. Tissue distribution of ACE2 protein, the functional receptor for SARS coronavirus. A first step in understanding SARS pathogenesis. J Pathol. 2004;203:631–7. https://doi.org/10.1002/path.1570.

58. Tai W, He L, Zhang X, et al. Characterization of the receptor-binding domain (RBD) of 2019 novel coronavirus: implication for development of RBD protein as a viral attachment inhibitor and vaccine. Cell Mol Immunol. 2020;17:613–20. https://doi.org/10.1038/s41423-020-0400-4.

59. Lau SK, Woo PC, Yip CC, et al. Coronavirus HKU1 and other coronavirus infections in Hong Kong. J Clin Microbiol. 2006;44(6):2063–71. https://doi.org/10.1128/JCM.02614-05.

60. MacNamara KC, Chua MM, Phillips JJ, et al. Contributions of the viral genetic background and a single amino acid substitution in an immunodominant CD8+ T-cell epitope to murine coronavirus neurovirulence. J Virol. 2005;79(14):9108–18. https://doi.org/10.1128/JVI.79.14.9108-9118.2005.

61. Mehta P, McAuley DF, Brown M, et al. HLH Across Speciality Collaboration, UK. COVID-19: consider cytokine storm syndromes and immunosuppression. Lancet. 2020;395(10229):1033–4. https://doi.org/10.1016/S0140-6736(20)30628-0.

62. Al-Olama M, Rashid A, Garozzo D. COVID-19-associated meningoencephalitis complicated with intracranial hemorrhage: a case report. Acta Neurochir. 2020;162(7):1495–9. https://doi.org/10.1007/s00701-020-04402-w.

63. Dogan L, Kaya D, Sarikaya T, et al. Plasmapheresis treatment in COVID-19-related autoimmune meningoencephalitis: case series. Brain Behav Immun. 2020;87:155–8. https://doi.org/10.1016/j.bbi.2020.05.022.

64. Piechotta V, Chai KL, Valk SJ, et al. Convalescent plasma or hyperimmune immunoglobulin for people with COVID-19: a living systematic review. Cochrane Database Syst Rev. 2020;7(7):CD013600. https://doi.org/10.1002/14651858.CD013600.pub2.

65. Zambreanu L, Lightbody S, Bhandari M, et al. A case of limbic encephalitis associated with asymptomatic COVID-19 infection. J Neurol Neurosurg Psychiatry. 2020;91:1229. https://doi.org/10.1136/jnnp-2020-323839.

66. Varatharaj A, Thomas N, Ellul MA, et al. Neurological and neuropsychiatric complications of COVID-19 in 153 patients: a UK-wide surveillance study. Lancet Psychiatry. 2020;7(10):875–82. https://doi.org/10.1016/S2215-0366(20)30287-X.

67. Xiong W, Mu J, Guo J, et al. New onset neurologic events in people with COVID-19 in 3 regions in China. Neurology. 2020;95(11):e1479–87. https://doi.org/10.1212/WNL.0000000000010034.

68. Pons-Escoda A, Naval-Baudín P, Majós C, et al. Neurologic Involvement in COVID-19: cause or coincidence? A neuroimaging perspective. AJNR Am J Neuroradiol. 2020;41(8):1365–9. https://doi.org/10.3174/ajnr.A6627.

69. Chougar L, Shor N, Weiss N, et al. CoCo Neurosciences study group. Retrospective observational study of brain magnetic resonance imaging findings in patients with acute SARS-CoV-2 infection and neurological manifestations. Radiology. 2020;297:E313. https://doi.org/10.1148/radiol.2020202422.

70. Montalvan V, Lee J, Bueso T, et al. Neurological manifestations of COVID-19 and other coronavirus infections: a systematic review. Clin Neurol Neurosurg. 2020;194:105921. https://doi.org/10.1016/j.clineuro.2020.105921.

71. Guilmot A, Maldonado Slootjes S, et al. Immune-mediated neurological syndromes in SARS-CoV-2-infected patients. J Neurol. 2020:1–7. https://doi.org/10.1007/s00415-020-10108-x.

72. Toscano G, Palmerini F, Ravaglia S, et al. Guillain-Barré syndrome associated with SARS-CoV-2. N Engl J Med. 2020;382(26):2574–6. https://doi.org/10.1056/NEJMc2009191.

73. Gutiérrez-Ortiz C, Méndez-Guerrero A, Rodrigo-Rey S, et al. Miller Fisher syndrome and polyneuritis cranialis in COVID-19. Neurology. 2020;95(5):e601–5. https://doi.org/10.1212/WNL.0000000000009619.

74. Pilotto A, Odolini S, Masciocchi S, et al. Steroid-responsive encephalitis in coronavirus disease 2019. Ann Neurol. 2020;88:423. https://doi.org/10.1002/ana.25783.

75. Scullen T, Keen J, Mathkour M, et al. Coronavirus 2019 (COVID-19)-associated encephalopathies and cerebrovascular disease: the New Orleans experience. World Neurosurg. 2020;141:e437–46. https://doi.org/10.1016/j.wneu.2020.05.192.

76. Zuhorn F, Omaimen H, Ruprecht B, et al. Parainfectious encephalitis in COVID-19: "The Claustrum Sign". J Neurol. 2020:1–4. https://doi.org/10.1007/s00415-020-10185-y.

77. Yoshikawa K, Kuwahara M, Morikawa M, et al. Varied antibody reactivities and clinical relevance in anti-GQ1b antibody-related diseases. Neurol Neuroimmunol Neuroinflamm. 2018;5(6):e501. https://doi.org/10.1212/NXI.0000000000000501.

78. Chi MS, Ng SH, Chan LY. Asymmetric acute motor axonal neuropathy with unilateral tongue swelling mimicking stroke. Neurologist. 2016;21(6):106–8. https://doi.org/10.1097/NRL.0000000000000102.

79. Hayashi M, Sahashi Y, Baba Y, et al. COVID-19-associated mild encephalitis/encephalopathy with a reversible splenial lesion. J Neurol Sci. 2020;415:116941. https://doi.org/10.1016/j.jns.2020.116941.

80. Wong PF, Craik S, Newman P, et al. Lessons of the month 1: a case of rhombencephalitis as a rare

complication of acute COVID-19 infection. Clin Med (Lond). 2020;20(3):293–4. https://doi.org/10.7861/clinmed.2020-0182.

81. Paterson RW, Brown RL, Benjamin L, et al. UCL Queen Square National Hospital for Neurology and Neurosurgery COVID-19 Study Group. The emerging spectrum of COVID-19 neurology: clinical, radiolog-ical and laboratory findings. Brain. 2020;143:3104. https://doi.org/10.1093/brain/awaa240.

82. Virhammar J, Kumlien E, Fällmar D, et al. Acute necrotizing encephalopathy with SARS-CoV-2 RNA confirmed in cerebrospinal fluid. Neurology. 2020;95(10):445–9. https://doi.org/10.1212/WNL.0000000000010250.

Possible Thrombotic Microangiopathy Occurring in Patient with CNS Localization of SARS-Cov-2

Simonetta Gerevini, Angela Napolitano,
Mariangela Cava, Emilio Giazzi,
and Cristina Agostinis

It is well documented that SARS-CoV-2 can cause damage to endothelial cells in the lungs, the heart, and the kidneys, activating inflammatory and thrombotic pathways [1]. Endothelial cell infection or monocyte activation, upregulation of tissue factors, and the release of microparticles, which activate the thrombotic pathway and cause microangiopathy, might occur for SARS-CoV-2 as for other viruses [2].

In COVID-19 pneumonia, the extensive microvascular damage seems to be related to a macrophage activation syndrome (MAS)-like mechanism [3] which differs from disseminated intravascular coagulopathy (DIC) and induces a coagulopathic cascade with subsequent local microthrombosis and microbleeding in the small pulmonary vessels. A similar immune-mediated microvascular damage could be responsible for CNS manifestations [4].

The binding of SARS-CoV-2 to angiotensin converting enzyme 2 (ACE2) is a critical step in the pathophysiology of clinical manifestations in patients with COVID-19 [5], as it triggers the formation of a cytokine storm, with marked elevation in the levels of interleukin-1, interleukin-6, and tumor necrosis factor [6]. High levels of these cytokines increase vascular permeability, edema, and widespread inflammation with consequent multiorgan damage [7]. ACE2 receptor is widely expressed on human cells in multiple organs, including blood vessels and the brain [8].

Thrombocytopenia with elevated D-dimer and C-reactive protein in severe COVID-19 and the high prevalence of thrombotic lesions in these patients are consistent with a virus-associated microangiopathic process. Endothelial dysfunction can potentially lead to microvascular and macrovascular complications in the brain, as described so far [9].

MRI signs of brain microvascular injury consists of small SWI hypointensities with a peculiar distribution; in particular corpus callosum is one of the more frequent location.

Extensive and isolated WM microhemorrhages pattern is also reported in critically ill patients, resulting from long term intubation or ECMO [10, 11]. These findings were recently described in a small number of critically ill patients with COVID-19 [12]. Nevertheless, only

S. Gerevini (✉) · C. Agostinis
Neuroradiology Department, Papa Giovanni XXIII Hospital, Bergamo, Italy
e-mail: sgerevini@asst-pg23.it;
agostinis@asst-pg23.it

A. Napolitano
Department of Clinical and Experimental Radiology, San Raffaele Scientific Institute, Milan, Italy
e-mail: napolitano.angela@hsr.it

M. Cava
Department of Radiology, ASL-AL San Giacomo Hospital, Novi Ligure, Italy

E. Giazzi
Department of Neuroradiology, ASST Papa Giovanni XXIII, Bergamo, Italy
e-mail: egiazzi@asst-pg23.it

a subgroup of our patients required ICU hospitalization.

Similar imaging findings are reported in severe acute respiratory distress syndromes [13], including high altitude cerebral edema (HACE) [14]. Interestingly, in these published cases, microbleeds in the corpus callosum are associated with a restriction on diffusion-weighted sequences, as for cytotoxic edema. The localization of the lesions is very similar to what observed in our series; however, in none of our patient there was associated edema nor focal neither diffuse brain swelling.

Stroke associated with a generalized thrombotic predisposition in COVID-19 is of particular interest. Four out of the eight patients had cardiovascular risk factors for stroke including atrial fibrillation. One patient had pulmonary emboli, but still the presence of microthrombi in the distal portions of the pulmonary vascular tree cannot be excluded. COVID-19 is associated with a prothrombotic state and highly elevated D-dimer levels, and abnormal coagulation parameters have been shown to be associated with poor outcome [15]. In our cohort we observed similar gross coagulation values, but an increased inflammatory response that could be linked with increased micro thrombotic events.

Cerebral microbleeds are usually due to extravasation of red blood cells, and in the context of COVID-19 could be due to endothelial dysfunction related to viral binding to the ACE-2 receptors expressed on endothelial cells. Indeed, a recent report described direct viral infection of the endothelial cell and diffuse endothelial inflammation in multiple organ systems [1].

Endothelial injury can occur in the smallest blood vessels and can be considered as "microangiopathy". Furthermore, activation of the complement related to the viral infection can determine microthrombi formation. We have also to consider that the term "thrombotic" indicates the presence of blood clots. We can speculate that microthrombotic or microangiopatic lesions can occur in other organs besides the lungs, as in the kidneys, the heart, and the brain at the level of the cerebral small vessels, as previously described [16–18].

SWI sequence can detect micro- and macro hemorrhages and delineate cerebral microvasculature and can also reveal low-flow vascular malformations; furthermore, it provides differentiation of calcium from hemorrhage in the brain. Oxyhemoglobin is diamagnetic in nature, whereas deoxyhemoglobin is paramagnetic. The paramagnetic deoxyhemoglobin serves as an intrinsic contrast agent on SWI sequences, and is low in signal. This causes magnetic field inhomogeneity due to two effects: a reduction of T2* and a phase difference between the vessel and its surrounding tissue. This property also forms the basic principle for blood oxygen level dependent functional and venographic imaging. This physical aspect of the SWI sequence can explain why the majority of focal T2 hypointensities are not seen on GE, also supporting the presence not of a true hemorrhage but at least of micro thrombosis, that can be located in the vessel wall rather than in the vessel lumen. These findings can be suspicious for endothelial microbleeds (EMBs)/ microthrombi.

A larger prospective study would be necessary to clarify if this pattern of susceptibility imaging abnormalities as observed in this subset of COVID-19 patients with neurological manifestations, may be related to a thrombotic microangiopathy. In this perspective, histopathological correlation could be enlightening.

5.1 Clinical Cases (Figs. 5.1, 5.2, 5.3, 5.4, 5.5, 5.6, 5.7, 5.8, 5.9 and 5.10)

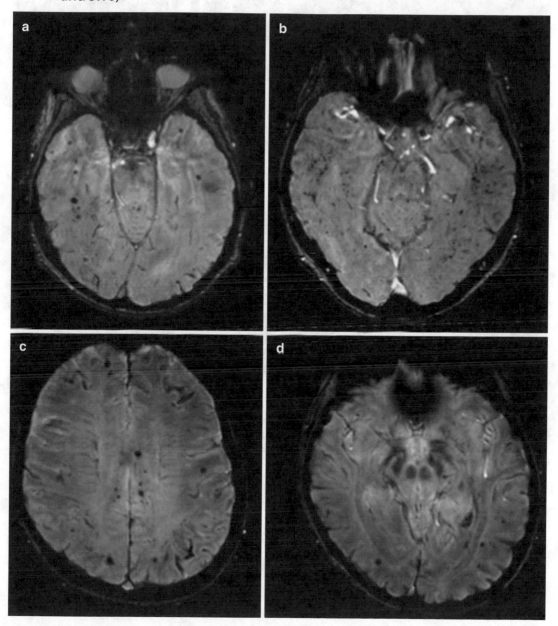

Fig. 5.1 Axial SWI images show multiple hypointense foci and their spread into lobes: temporal (Panels **a**, **b**), frontal, occipital, and temporal in the same patient (Panels **c**, **d**)

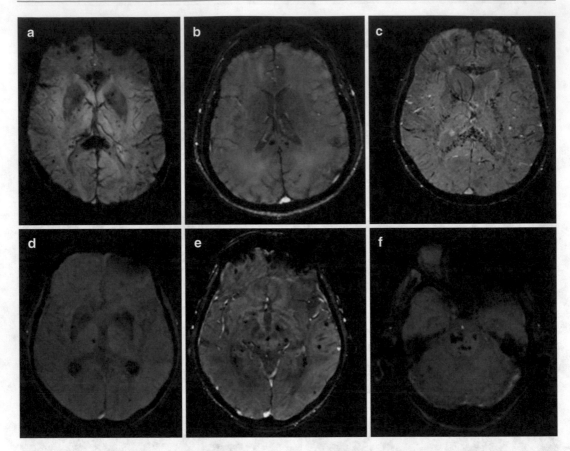

Fig. 5.2 SWI images show multiple hypointense foci with more diffuse lesions in the splenium and genu of the corpus callosum as the more consistently involved structure (**a**, **b**), diffuse punctate hypointensities at the level of internal capsule (Panel **c**) somehow depicting the perivascular spaces. Panel (**d**) shows hypointense foci on axial SWI images at thalamic level. SWI images at posterior fossa and the level of basal cisterns demonstrate diffuse hemorrhagic foci predominantly involving the brainstem (Panels **e**, **f**)

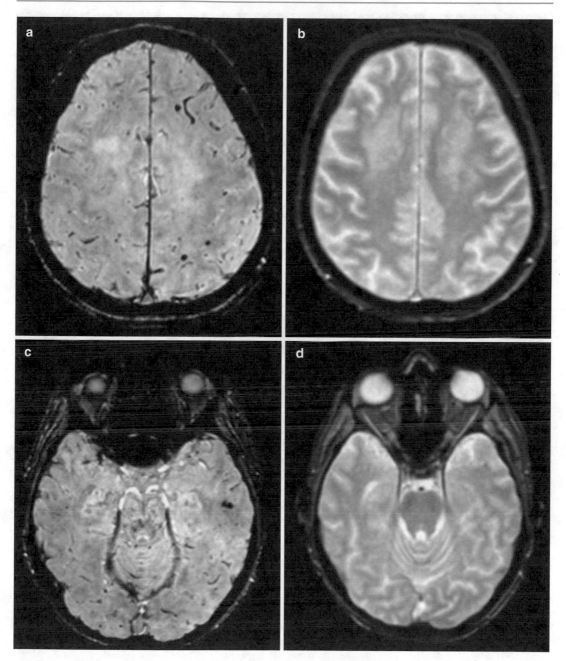

Fig. 5.3 The comparison between images acquired in the SWI (**a**, **c**) and GE sequences (**b**, **d**) at the same levels demonstrates the best diagnostic performance of the for-mer in the detection of micro thrombotic/micro hemor-rhagic hypointense foci

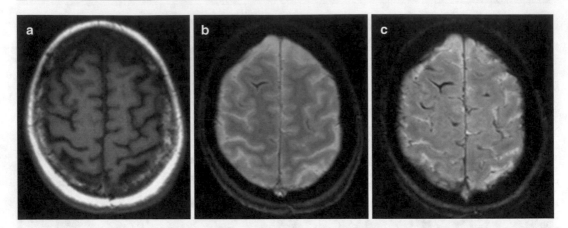

Fig. 5.4 Images acquired in T1 (**a**), GE and SWI sequences (**b**, **c**) at the same level shows absence of signal alteration, micro hemorrhagic hypointense foci and linear cortical hemorrhagic images in T1-s compared to the other two sequences

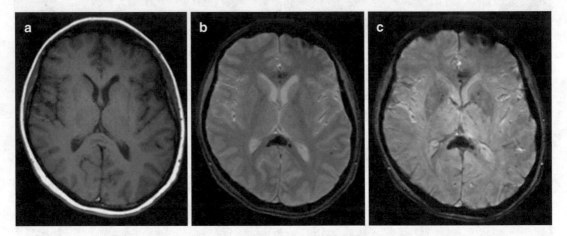

Fig. 5.5 Images acquired in GE and SWI sequences (**b**, **c**) at the same level show severely hypointense cluster of lesions in the splenium and genu of the corpus callosum, which corresponds to nonsignificant alteration of the signal intensity in the T1 (**a**) sequence

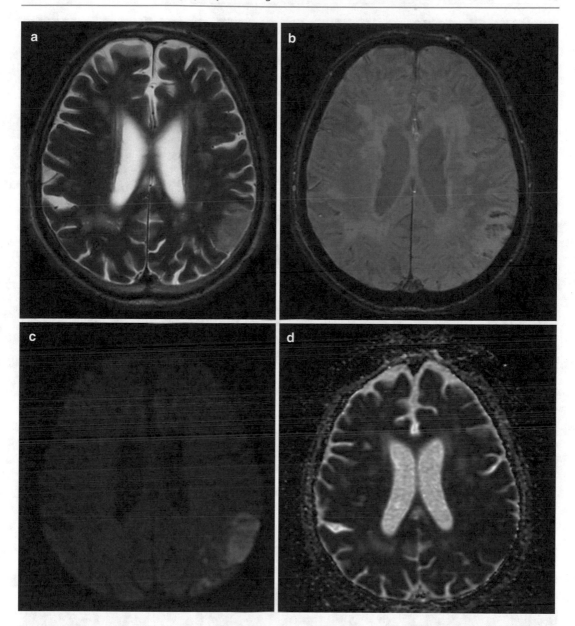

Fig. 5.6 The panel describes a type of lesion frequently observed in COVID patients, with typical appearance of left parietal cortico-subcortical ischemic lesion, evident as hyperintensity in T2 (**a**) and DWI sequences at high values of B (**b**), with restriction and hypointensity at ADC map (**d**); also in this area, focal hypointense spots can be observed in the gradient echo sequences, probably indicative of thrombotic / haemorrhagic phenomena (**c**)

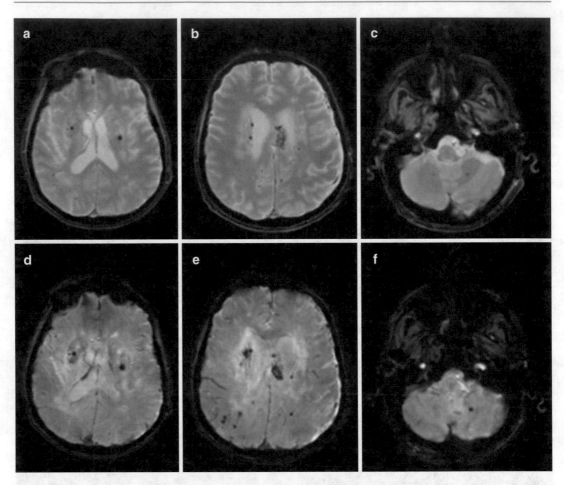

Fig. 5.7 (**a–c**) Panel shows hypointense foci repr esent-ing microthrombotic / microhemorrhagic lesions in supra-tentoril and subtentorial areas, confirming them as better detectable in SWI sequences (**d–f**) compared to GE con-ventional imaging (**a–c**)

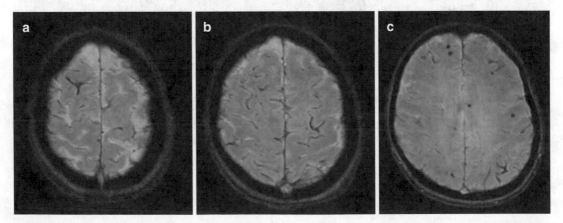

Fig. 5.8 Patient presenting at the same time and at differ-ent levels the concomitant presence of microhemorrhagic / microthrombotic lesions represented by hypointensity foci (**c**) and subarachnoid hypointense striae adjacent to sulci, which delineate more extensive and non-focal hemorrhagic areas (**a–c**)

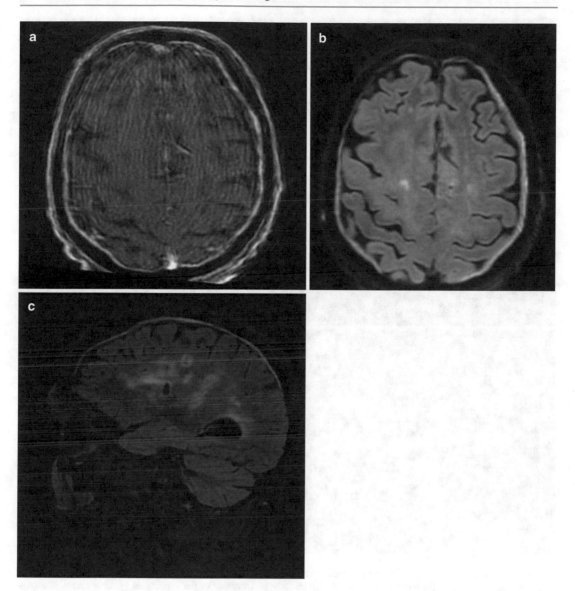

Fig. 5.9 Patient presenting marked ubiquitous meningeal thickening especially in the fronto-parieto-occipital site, clearly evident in the FLAIR sequences (**b**, **c**) and characterized by intense enhancement after gadolinium infusion (**a**)

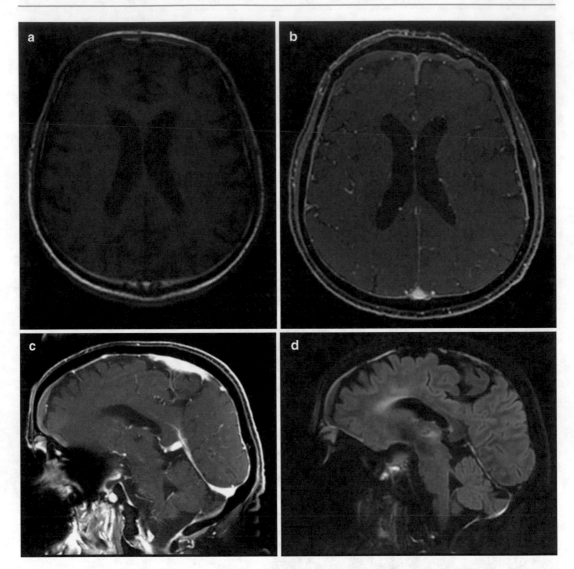

Fig. 5.10 Patient presenting diffused meningeal thickening in supratentorial and subtentorial areas, outlined by enhancement in the sequences acquired after contrast medium infusion (**b, d**), especially in comparison with the image acquired in precontrast T1s (**a**); a thickening and hyperintensity of the meningeal plane is also well recognizable in the FLAIR sequence (**c**)

Acknowledgments Pastorino Roberto MD, Department of Radiology, ASL-AL San Giacomo Hospital, Novi Ligure, Italy

References

1. Varga Z, Flammer AJ, Steiger P, Haberecker M, Andermatt R, Zinkernagel AS, Mehra MR, Schuepbach RA, Ruschitzka F, Moch H. Endothelial cell infection and endotheliitis in COVID-19. Lancet. 2020;395:1417–8.

2. Brisse E, Wouters CH, Andrei G, Matthys P. How viruses contribute to the pathogenesis of hemophagocytic lymphohistiocytosis. Front Immunol. 2017;8:1102.
3. McGonagle D, O'Donnell JS, Sharif K, Emery P, Bridgewood C. Immune mechanisms of pulmonary intravascular coagulopathy in COVID-19 pneumonia. Lancet Rheumatol. 2020;2:e437–45.
4. Needham EJ, Chou SH-Y, Coles AJ, Menon DK. Neurological implications of COVID-19 infections. Neurocrit Care. 2020;32:667. https://doi.org/10.1007/s12028-020-00978-4.
5. Verdecchia P, Cavallini C, Spanevello A, Angeli F. The pivotal link between ACE2 deficiency and

SARS-CoV-2 infection. Eur J Intern Med. 2020;76: 14–20.

6. Mehta P, McAuley DF, Brown M, Sanchez E, Tattersall RS, Manson JJ. COVID-19: consider cytokine storm syndromes and immunosuppression. Lancet. 2020;395:1033–4.

7. Chen G, Wu D, Guo W, et al. Clinical and immunological features of severe and moderate coronavirus disease 2019. J Clin Invest. 2020;130:2620–9.

8. Baig AM, Khaleeq A, Ali U, Syeda H. Evidence of the COVID-19 virus targeting the CNS: tissue distribution, host–virus interaction, and proposed neurotropic mechanisms. ACS Chem Neurosci. 2020;11: 995–8.

9. Klok FA, Kruip MJHA, van der Meer NJM, et al. Incidence of thrombotic complications in critically ill ICU patients with COVID-19. Thromb Res. 2020;191:145–7.

10. Fanou EM, Coutinho JM, Shannon P, Kiehl TR, Levi MM, Wilcox ME, Aviv RI, Mandell DM. Critical illness-associated cerebral microbleeds. Stroke. 2017;48:1085–7.

11. Liebeskind DS, Sanossian N, Sapo ML, Saver JL. Cerebral microbleeds after use of extracorporeal membrane oxygenation in children. J Neuroimaging. 2013;23:75–8.

12. Radmanesh A, Derman A, Lui YW, Raz E, Loh JP, Hagiwara M, Borja MJ, Zan E, Fatterpekar GM. COVID-19–associated diffuse leukoencephalopathy and microhemorrhages. Radiology. 2020;297:E223.

13. Riech S, Kallenberg K, Moerer O, Hellen P, Bärtsch P, Quintel M, Knauth M. The pattern of brain microhemorrhages after severe lung failure resembles the one seen in high-altitude cerebral edema. Crit Care Med. 2015;43:e386.

14. Hackett PH, Yarnell PR, Weiland DA, Reynard KB. Acute and evolving MRI of high-altitude cerebral edema: microbleeds, edema, and pathophysiology. Am J Neuroradiol. 2019;40:464–9.

15. Tang N, Li D, Wang X, Sun Z. Abnormal coagulation parameters are associated with poor prognosis in patients with novel coronavirus pneumonia. J Thromb Haemost. 2020;18:844–7.

16. Magro C, Mulvey JJ, Berlin D, Nuovo G, Salvatore S, Harp J, Baxter-Stoltzfus A, Laurence J. Complement associated microvascular injury and thrombosis in the pathogenesis of severe COVID-19 infection: a report of five cases. Transl Res. 2020:1–13.

17. Coolen T, Lolli V, Sadeghi N, et al. Early postmortem brain MRI findings in COVID-19 non-survivors. Neurology. 2020;95:e2016.

18. Noris M, Benigni A, Remuzzi G. The case of complement activation in COVID-19 multiorgan impact. Kidney Int. 2020;98:314–22.

Still to Be Explored: Involvement of Other Districts/Organs in COVID-19 Patients

6

Simonetta Gerevini

At the start of the pandemic in February–March, 2020, COVID-19 patients were mainly affected by pulmonary disease with diffuse alveolar damage in severe cases. In Chapters 7, 8 and 9 the authors want to open a window with some pills on other possible manifestation of this virus, still not completely well known.

Involvement of other organs has been suggested in patients with systemic and severe progressive disease who have cardiac, neurological, and gastrointestinal symptoms and we will see some of this possible spectrum.

Endotheliitis and thrombosis in patients with COVID-19 are proved by the high rate of observed thromboembolic events. Rapidly accumulating body of evidence suggests that COVID-19 causes vascular derangements as a consequence of endothelial cell infection by the virus, but pathological mechanisms have to be fully clarified. Furthermore, toxic and inflammatory systemic reaction to the virus is not completely understood as well as the effect of this reaction on various organs.

In Chap. 7 we will show some preliminary neuroradiological findings in a small cohort of COVID-19 positive neonates. Furthermore, histopathological findings are briefly described in both heart (Chap. 8) and brain (Chap. 9) of COVID-19 patients.

S. Gerevini (✉)
Neuroradiology Department, Papa Giovanni XXIII
Hospital, Bergamo, Italy
e-mail: sgerevini@asst-pg23.it

S. Gerevini (ed.), *Neuroimaging of Covid-19. First Insights based on Clinical Cases*,
https://doi.org/10.1007/978-3-030-67521-9_6

Brain Imaging Findings in COVID-19 Positive Newborns

7

Ornella Manara, Antonino Barletta,
Giulio Pezzetti, and Simonetta Gerevini

7.1   Introduction

Only limited data regarding COVID-19 infection in paediatric and neonatal population are available yet: COVID-19 tends to spare newborns and risk of severe disease in infected patients is low [1].

A retrospective review of 1099 cases of COVID-19 in China identified nine children [2] and, according to a retrospective study of 266 hospitalized children in Wuhan, the virus was isolated in only six children [range 1–7 years age]: only one child had severe disease requiring intensive care [3]. After an outbreak of Kawasaki disease in paediatric patients, some colleagues from our hospital in Bergamo, have suggested in a recent work that also children can be affected by SARS-CoV-2 even if not directly for pulmonary involvement at least with endothelial damage. Moreover, SARS-CoV-2 epidemic was associated with high incidence of a severe form of Kawasaki disease [4].

About newborns, since SARS-CoV-2 is contained in most body fluids and secretions, faecal-oral transmission can occur, raising the possibility of transmission from mother to baby at birth, although not prenatally.

Few data on CNS involvement by COVID-19 infection in paediatric and neonatal population are reported in the literature [5, 6]: in a study of children with respiratory disease and acute encephalitis-like syndrome, in approximately 12% of cases there was evidence of an acute coronavirus infection [7].

Few reports of encephalitis [8] including Bickerstaff's encephalitis [9] are available regarding MERS: MRI showed hyperintense signal abnormalities on T2-weighted imaging in deep and subcortical white matter, corpus callosum and basal ganglia [8].

In a 5-year-old child with lower extremity pain, impaired walking, peripheral facial weakness and bulbar palsy, HCoV-OC43 infection has been found [8]. MERS can also trigger a post-infectious brainstem encephalitis and Guillain-Barre syndrome [10]. Regarding COVID-19, there are Chinese reports of transverse myelitis [11].

There are three main ways in which COVID-19 could affect newborns:

1. Newborns might be infected by COVID-19 before, during or soon after birth: this may lead to breathing or feeding problems, requiring hospitalization.
2. COVID-19 could affect newborns already hospitalized for other medical conditions (like prematurity) that increase the risk of severe infection.

O. Manara · A. Barletta · G. Pezzetti · S. Gerevini (✉)
Neuroradiology Department, Papa Giovanni XXIII Hospital, Bergamo, Italy
e-mail: omanara@asst-pg23.it; abarletta@asst-pg23.it; gpezzetti@asst-pg23.it; sgerevini@asst-pg23.it

© The Author(s), under exclusive license to Springer Nature Switzerland AG 2021
S. Gerevini (ed.), *Neuroimaging of Covid-19. First Insights based on Clinical Cases*,
https://doi.org/10.1007/978-3-030-67521-9_7

83

3. COVID-19 can modify the clinical management of mothers during pregnancy or labour, leading to indirect problems to some babies although not directly infected by the virus [1].

7.2   Case Description

Between February and May 2020, seven all term neonates with adequate Apgar score (age range 44–118 days, average 81 days; three males and four females) were evaluated at the Neonatal Intensive Care or Sub-Intensive Care Unit and Neuroradiology Department of our hospital (Papa Giovanni XXIII Hospital in Bergamo, Italy), mainly due to fever and feeding impairment. All patients had a positive swab therefore they were considered as proved cases of SARS-CoV-2 infection and hospitalized in COVID-19 dedicated wards. Only three mothers had a positive SARS-CoV-2 nasopharyngeal swab at the NICU admission of their babies: mothers weren't tested for COVID-19 at the time of labour.

The medium age of nasopharyngeal swab normalization was 38.5 days.

7.2.1   Magnetic Resonance Imaging (MRI)

In all patients, no morphologic anomalies nor qualitative and quantitative signal alterations in grey and white matter on all the sequences performed in particular on T1 and T2-w sequences (data not shown).

In four cases (patients 3, 4, 5, 7) we visually found a mild to moderate reduced diffusion in the genu of the corpus callosum (hyperintensity in DWI and hypo intensity on the ADC map): this finding was confirmed on quantitative ROI-based (see methods) analysis of the genu of the corpus callosum (example of patient 4 in Fig. 7.1).

ADC and FA values were compared to normal ones (corrected for age) reported in the literature [12–17].

Regarding the splenium of the corpus callosum, no signal alterations on DWI were found at visual inspection: quantitative ADC ROI analysis

revealed mild diffusion reduction compared to the literature, especially in patient 2.

In six out of the seven COVID-19 neonates, there was a mild diffusion reduction in the genu of the corpus callosum. In five cases restriction can be appreciated both on visual inspection and with a quantitative analysis while in one case only ROI-based approach was able to highlight this finding. Only by quantitative assessment a slight diffusion restriction in the splenium of the corpus callosum can be picked up. FA and T1-T2 signal were in normal ranges in the corpus callosum.

Well-known entities associated with involvement of the splenium of the corpus callosum include the reversible splenial lesion syndrome (RESLES) and MERS, which is a clinical-radiological entity characterized by mild encephalitis or encephalopathy associated with reversible lesion of the splenium of the corpus callosum. Transient lesions in the splenium of the corpus callosum can occur in several conditions such as epilepsy, following the sudden withdrawal of antiepileptic drugs, influenza encephalitis, and other conditions such as haemolytic-uremic syndrome, subarachnoid haemorrhage, trauma (diffuse axonal injury), hypoglycaemia, hypernatremia, osmotic myelinolysis, Wernicke encephalopathy, Marchiafava–Bignami disease and haemolytic-uremic syndrome [18–20].

In addition, isolated involvement of the splenium of the corpus callosum may also occur in patients with ADEM [21]. We can consider that the lesion in the splenium of the corpus callosum in our patients is of demyelinating nature (likely post-viral).

The pathogenesis can be related to markedly increased levels of cytokines and extracellular glutamate, leading to dysfunction of the callosal neurons and microglia. Cytotoxic oedema develops when water becomes trapped in these cells [18, 19].

Cytotoxic lesions of the corpus callosum (CLOCCs) are areas of low diffusion, equal or slightly low T1 signal, high signal on T2-FLAIR sequences and no enhancement after paramagnetic contrast agent injection. It is also possible to observe only diffusion reduction without any

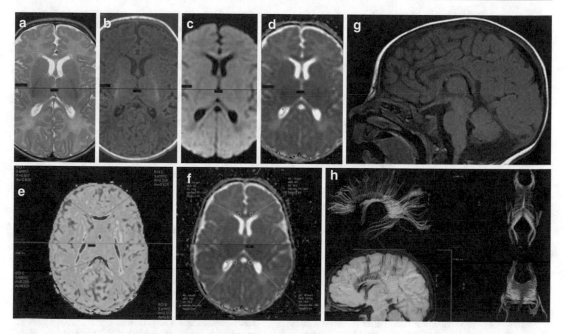

Fig. 7.1 Qualitative and quantitative assessment of the genu and splenium of the corpus callosum in patient 4 (the most significant) on morphologic, diffusion and diffusion-tensor imaging. (**a, b, g**): T2-weighted and T1 weighted (3D Ax T1 and Sag SE T1) sequence for genu and splenium of the corpus callosum (separated enlarged view). (**c, d**): DWI and ADC with diffusion restriction in the genu of the corpus callosum. (**e, f**): Quantitative ROI-based evaluation of corpus callosum on coloured FA and ADC map, respectively, in which an ADC reduction and mild FA increase compared to the literature can been appreciated (see text). (**h**): DTI reconstruction of corpus callosum (deterministic tractography) with normal findings

abnormal signals under conventional sequences. These lesions tend to be midline and relatively symmetric [18–22].

Viral aetiologies represent the most common cause of CLOCCs callosal lesions, which usually become evident from as early as 2 day of onset of symptoms. Among all the possible viral agents (influenza, rotavirus, mumps, *E. coli*, adenovirus), rotavirus and Parechovirus have peculiar imaging pattern [18, 22, 23]. To date, both in adult and in paediatric/neonatal population, no cases of selective genu involvement have been described [18–22].

Then, our findings of selective moderate diffusion reduction in the genu (and, in a lesser extent, in the splenium) of the corpus callosum might represent a different type of CLOCCs possibly related to COVID-19 CNS neonatal infection. Larger studies are needed to confirm and better understand these findings and the appearance of these data in this atlas is just to be aware of these possible findings.

References

1. Tezer H, Bedir Demirdag T. Novel coronavirus disease (COVID-19) in children. Turk J Med Sci. 2020;50:592–603. https://doi.org/10.3906/sag-2004-174.
2. Guan W, Ni ZY, Hu Y, et al. Clinical characteristics of coronavirus disease 2019 in China. N Engl J Med. 2020;382(18):1708–20. https://doi.org/10.1056/NEJMoa2002032.
3. Liu W, Zhang Q, Chen J, et al. Detection of Covid-19 in children in early January 2020 in Wuhan, China. N Engl J Med. 2020;382:1370–1. https://doi.org/10.1056/NEJMc2003717.
4. Verdoni L, Mazza A, Gervasoni A, et al. An outbreak of severe Kawasaki-like disease at the Italian Epicentre of the SARS-CoV-2 epidemic: an observational cohort study. Lancet. 2020;395(10239):1771–8. https://doi.org/10.1016/S0140-6736(20)31103-X.
5. Zhu H, Wang L, Fang C, et al. Clinical analysis of 10 neonates born from mothers with 2019-nCoV pneumonia. Transl Pediatr. 2020;9(1):51–60. https://doi.org/10.21037/tp.2020.02.06.
6. Chen H, Guo J, Wang C, et al. Clinical characteristics and intrauterine vertical transmission potential of COVID-19 infection in nine pregnant women:

a retrospective review of medical records. Lancet. 2020;395(10226):809–15. https://doi.org/10.1016/S0140-6736(20)30360-3.

7. Li Y, Li H, Fan R, et al. Coronavirus Infections in the Central Nervous System and Respiratory Tract Show Distinct Features in Hospitalized Children. Intervirology. 2016;59:163–9. https://doi.org/10.1159/000453066.

8. Arabi YM, Harthi A, Hussein J. Severe neurologic syndrome associated with Middle East respiratory syndrome corona virus (MERS-CoV). Infection. 2015;43(4):495–501. https://doi.org/10.1007/s15010-015-0720-y.

9. Kim JE, Heo JH, Kim H. Neurological complications during treatment of middle east respiratory syndrome. J Clin Neurol. 2017;13(3):227–33. https://doi.org/10.3988/jcn.2017.13.3.227.

10. Sharma K, Tengsupakul S, Sanchez O. Guillain–Barré syndrome with unilateral peripheral facial and bulbar palsy in a child: a case report. SAGE Open Med Case Rep. 2019;7:1–5. https://doi.org/10.1177/2050313X19838750.

11. Wang D, Hu B, Hu C, et al. Clinical characteristics of 138 hospitalized patients with 2019 novel coronavirus-infected pneumonia in Wuhan, China. JAMA. 2020;323(11):1061–9. https://doi.org/10.1001/jama.2020.1585.

12. Zhang L, Thomas KM, Davidson MC, et al. MR quantitation of volume and diffusion changes in the developing brain. AJNR Am J Neuroradiol. 2005;26:45–9.

13. Provenzale JM, Isaacson J, Chen S. Progression of corpus callosum diffusion-tensor imaging values during a period of signal changes consistent with myelination. AJR Am J Roentgenol. 2012;198:1403–8. https://doi.org/10.2214/AJR.11.7849.

14. Engelbrecht V, Scherer A, Rassek M, et al. Diffusion-weighted MR imaging in the brain in children: findings in the normal brain and in the brain with white matter diseases. Radiology. 2002;222:410–8. https://doi.org/10.1148/radiol.2222010492.

15. Groenendaal F. Diffusion of the corpus callosum in young infants. Lett Ed Neuropediatr. 2016;50(6):411. https://doi.org/10.1055/s-0039-1694987.

16. Hasegawa T, Yamada K, Morimoto M. Development of corpus callosum in preterm infants is affected by the prematurity: in vivo assessment of diffusion tensor imaging at term-equivalent age. Pediatr Res. 2011;69(3):249–54. https://doi.org/10.1203/PDR.0b013e3182084e54.

17. Zhai G, Lin W, Wilber KP. Comparisons of regional white matter diffusion in healthy neonates and adults performed with a 3.0-T head-only MR imaging unit. Radiology. 2003;229:673–81. https://doi.org/10.1148/radiol.2293021462.

18. Starkey J, Kobayashi N, Numaguchi Y, et al. Cytotoxic lesions of the corpus callosum that show restricted diffusion: mechanisms, causes and manifestations. Radiographics. 2017;37:562–76. https://doi.org/10.1148/rg.2017160085.

19. Kazi AZ, Joshi PC, Kelkar AB. MRI evaluation of pathologies affecting the corpus callosum: a pictorial essay. Indian J Radiol Imag. 2013;23(4):321–32. https://doi.org/10.4103/0971-3026.125604.

20. Park SE, Choi DS, Shin HS, et al. Splenial lesions of the corpus callosum: disease spectrum and MRI findings. Korean J Radiol. 2017;18:710–21. https://doi.org/10.3348/kjr.2017.18.4.710.

21. Blaauw J, Meiners LC. The splenium of the corpus callosum: embryology, anatomy, function and imaging with pathophysiological hypothesis. Neuroradiology. 2020;62:563–85. https://doi.org/10.1007/s00234-019-02357-z.

22. Li G, Li S, Qi F. Mild encephalitis/encephalopathy in children with a reversible splenial lesion. Radiol Infect Dis. 2018;5:118e122.

Cardiac Involvement in COVID-19 Infection

Cardiac Involvement in COVID-19 Infection

Giulio Guagliumi, Dario Pellegrini, Aloke Finn, and Simonetta Gerevini

COVID-19 infection appeared to be associated with increased risk of thrombotic events, ranging from microvascular thrombosis to venous thromboembolic disease (including deep vein thrombosis and pulmonary embolism), and stroke [1].

Such thrombotic manifestations could be associated with multiorgan failure and increased mortality observed in a significant portion of patients, and suggest the presence of an underlying hypercoagulable status. Causes are still unclear, although cytokine storm and hyperactivation of complement-mediated immune response and endothelial damage have been proposed as possible mechanisms. Indeed, SARS-CoV-2 may be able to invade endothelial cells through angiotensin-converting enzyme 2 (ACE-2) and TMPRSS2 (transmembrane serine protease 2), which are highly expressed on the endothelial cell surface, and lead to inflammation in the endothelium [2].

Lymphocytic endotheliitis with recruitment of inflammatory cells was observed in the lungs, heart, liver and kidneys [2] on histological assessment, although prevalence of infection and viral-related extrapulmonary damage showed significant variability across published reports [3].

Systemic anticoagulation was associated with prolonged survival in patients hospitalized with COVID-19 [4] although uncertainty persists on best drug and dose choice, both in terms of efficacy and safety.

8.1 Cardiac Involvement

A broad spectrum of cardiovascular disorders have been reported in the setting of SARS-CoV-2, including acute coronary syndromes, myocardial injury and arrhythmias [5–7]. Acute myocardial injury, as evidenced by elevated levels of cardiac biomarkers or electrocardiogram abnormalities, was observed in 7–20% of pts. Children with COVID-19 have also been reported to develop hyperinflammatory shock with features similar to Kawasaki disease, including cardiac dysfunction and coronary vessel abnormalities. Direct viral invasion [8–11] and damage stemming from hyperimmune systemic reaction [9, 12–14] have been advanced as possible mechanisms, as inflammation and myocardial localization of coronavirus particles were described at endomyocardial biopsy.

G. Guagliumi · D. Pellegrini
Interventional Cardiology, Ospedale Papa Giovanni XXIII, Bergamo, Italy
e-mail: gguagliumi@asst-pg23.it; dpellegrini@asst-pg23.it

A. Finn
CVPath Institute, Gaithersburg, MD, USA
e-mail: afinn@cvpath.org

S. Gerevini (✉)
Neuroradiology Department, Papa Giovanni XXIII Hospital, Bergamo, Italy
e-mail: sgerevini@asst-pg23.it

© The Author(s), under exclusive license to Springer Nature Switzerland AG 2021
S. Gerevini (ed.), *Neuroimaging of Covid-19. First Insights based on Clinical Cases*,
https://doi.org/10.1007/978-3-030-67521-9_8

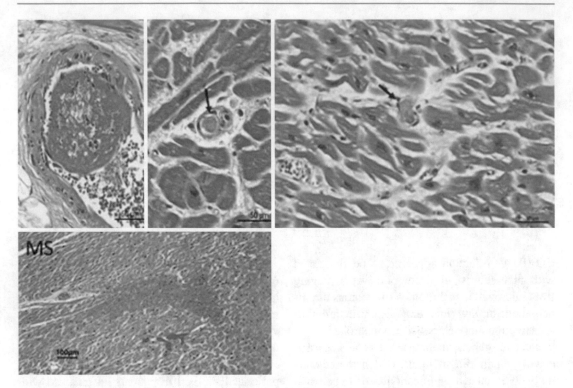

Fig. 8.1 Microthrombi as frequent cause of myocardial Injury observed in SARS-CoV-2 infection. Left ventricular microcirculation (capillaries and terminal arterioles) with presence of multiple Microthrombi (three different level of magnification) with surrounding areas of patchy myocardial injury

However, these findings suffered from high variability in published literature [15].

Acute coronary syndromes may be triggered different mechanisms, including the aforementioned hypercoagulable status, plaque rupture or spasm of epicardial coronary arteries [16, 17].

Recently, the pathologic finding of extensive thrombosis in the cardiac microcirculation has been described in a case of a young woman dying of ST-segment elevation acute myocardial infarction (STEMI), with normal coronary angiography [18]. No specific exams can detect microthrombi, so this phenomenon may explain the high number of reported acute coronary syndromes or acute myocardial dysfunction without a clear culprit lesion at angiography, which were at first deemed to be related to myocarditis. Finally, as similar thrombotic formations were reported also in the vascular bed of other extracardiac organs, this mechanism may be a specific feature of COVID-19, and may underlie the high rate of multiorgan failure. Hypercoagulable state, endothelial damage, cytokine storm and hyperactivation of macrophages have been postulated as possible mechanisms, but additional evidence is needed (Fig. 8.1) [19].

References

1. Nishiga M, Wang DW, Han Y, Lewis DB, Wu JC. COVID-19 and cardiovascular disease: from basic mechanisms to clinical perspectives. Nat Rev Cardiol. 2020;17:543–58.
2. Varga Z, Flammer A, Steiger P. Covid-19 endothelitis. Lancet. 2020;395:1417–8
3. Jayarangaiah A, Kariyanna PT, Chen X, Jayarangaiah A, Kumar A. COVID-19-Associated coagulopathy: an exacerbated immunothrombosis response. Clin Appl Thromb. 2020;26:1076029620943293. https://doi.org/10.1177/1076029620943293.
4. Paranjpe I, Fuster V, Lala A, et al. Association of treatment dose anticoagulation with in-hospital survival among hospitalized patients with COVID-19. J Am Coll Cardiol. 2020;76:122–4.
5. Shi S, Qin M, Shen B, et al. Association of cardiac injury with mortality in hospitalized patients

with COVID-19 in Wuhan, China. JAMA Cardiol. 2020;5:802.

6. Guo T, Fan Y, Chen M, Wu X, Zhang L, He T, Wang H, Wan J, Wang X, Lu Z. Cardiovascular implications of fatal outcomes of patients with coronavirus disease 2019 (COVID-19). JAMA Cardiol. 2020;5:811–8.

7. Shi S, Qin M, Cai Y, et al. Characteristics and clinical significance of myocardial injury in patients with severe coronavirus disease 2019. Eur Heart J. 2020;41:2070–9.

8. Hoffmann M, Kleine-Weber H, Schroeder S, et al. SARS-CoV-2 cell entry depends on ACE2 and TMPRSS2 and is blocked by a clinically proven protease inhibitor. Cell. 2020;181:271–280.e8.

9. Madjid M, Safavi-Naeini P, Solomon SD, Vardeny O. Potential effects of coronaviruses on the cardiovascular system: a review. JAMA Cardiol. 2020;5:831.

10. Li SSL, Cheng CW, Fu CL, Chan YH, Lee MP, Chan JWM, Yiu SF. Left ventricular performance in patients with severe acute respiratory syndrome: a 30-day echocardiographic follow-up study. Circulation. 2003;108:1798–803.

11. Tavazzi G, Pellegrini C, Maurelli M, et al. Myocardial localization of coronavirus in COVID-19 cardiogenic shock. Eur J Heart Fail. 2020;22:911–5.

12. Tay MZ, Poh CM, Rénia L, MacAry PA, Ng LFP. The trinity of COVID-19: immunity, inflammation and intervention. Nat Rev Immunol. 2020;20:363–74.

13. Driggin E, Madhavan MV, Bikdeli B, et al. Cardiovascular considerations for patients, health care workers, and health systems during the COVID-19 pandemic. J Am Coll Cardiol. 2020;75:2352–71.

14. Clerkin KJ, Fried JA, Raikhelkar J, et al. Coronavirus disease 2019 (COVID-19) and cardiovascular disease. Circulation. 2020;141:1648.

15. Lang JP, Wang X, Moura FA, Siddiqi HK, Morrow DA, Bohula EA. A current review of COVID-19 for the cardiovascular specialist. Am Heart J. 2020;226:29–44.

16. Libby P, Tabas I, Fredman G, Fisher EA. Inflammation and its resolution as determinants of acute coronary syndromes. Circ Res. 2014;114:1867–79

17. Bentzon JF, Otsuka F, Virmani R, Falk E. Mechanisms of plaque formation and rupture. Circ Res. 2014;114:1852–66.

18. Guagliumi G, Sonzogni A, Pescetelli I, Pellegrini D, Finn AV. Microthrombi and ST-segment-elevation myocardial infarction in COVID-19. Circulation. 2020;142:804–9.

19. Ackermann M, Verleden SE, Kuehnel M, et al. Pulmonary vascular endothelialitis, thrombosis, and angiogenesis in Covid-19. N Engl J Med. 2020;383:120–8. https://doi.org/10.1056/nejmoa2015432.

The Neuropathology Spectrum in Deceased Patients with COVID-19

9

Eleonora Aronica and Simonetta Gerevini

There is an increasing evidence of neurological and psychiatric manifestations in patients with COVID-19 [1, 2]. Recent postmortem studies reported a large spectrum of neuropathological features that support the neuro-invasive potential of SARS-CoV-2 [3–5]. Given the complex pathophysiology of COVID-19 associated neurological manifestation, the pathological changes observed at postmortem examination often reflect the combination of both direct and indirect cytopathic effects mediated by the virus, as well as of nonspecific complications of severe disease in the deceased patients with COVID-19 (i.e. critical illness-related encephalopathy [6]; and/or pre-existing medical conditions). Thus, all these factors need to be considered when interpreting neuropathological findings [3, 7]. Hypoxia-ischemia, observed in the majority of critically ill cases of Covid-19, does not account for all relevant neuropathological observations provided by postmortem neuropathological studies in single cases or small patient cohorts [8–14]. However, among these studies the extent and significance of neuroinflammatory changes associated with SARS-CoV-2 infection are still matter of discussion, with often contradictory conclusions. In particular, it remains unclear to what extent the reported microglia activation and occasionally the presence of sparse lymphocytic infiltrates (T lymphocytes) represents COVID-19-specific findings [6, 7].

In an autopsy cohort study performed in the Netherlands, detailed neuropathological examination was performed in 8 of 21 patients with full body autopsies and showed but only sparse T lymphocytes in parenchyma, but massive activation of microglia with microglial nodules, especially in the olfactory bulbs and brainstem ([15]; Fig. 9.1d–n). Given the regional heterogeneity and phenotypes of human microglia [16], whether microglia activated belongs to a specific subtype certainly deserves further attention, particularly in relation to the pattern of regional vulnerability observed in the context of a COVID-19 infection. Additionally, there is also evidence of increased blood–brain barrier (BBB) permeability (e.g. albumin extravasation, and its uptake in astrocytes; Fig. 9.1m). Understanding the association of neurological conditions in patients with SARS-CoV-2 infection with BBB dysfunction, particularly dissecting the underlying direct or indirect mechanisms, is worthy of future investigation [17].

E. Aronica
Department of (Neuro) Pathology, Amsterdam UMC, Neuroscience, Amsterdam, University of Amsterdam, Amsterdam, The Netherlands

Stichting Epilepsie Instellingen Nederland (SEIN), Heemstede, The Netherlands
e-mail: e.aronica@amsterdamumc.nl

S. Gerevini (✉)
Neuroradiology Department, Papa Giovanni XXIII Hospital, Bergamo, Italy
e-mail: sgerevini@asst-pg23.it

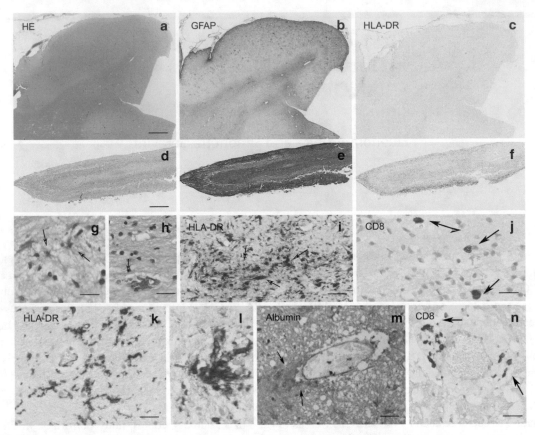

Fig. 9.1 Common neuropathological findings in deceased patients with COVID-19. Case: A 73-year-old male admitted to the intensive care (IC) unit with respiratory failure due to SARS-CoV-2 infection. Death occurred within 10 days (respiratory insufficiency due to viral pneumonia). (**a–c**): Frontal cortex (**a**, HE) showing reactive astrogliosis (**b**, GFAP), but not evident activation of the microglia (HLA-DR, **c**). (**d–j**): Olfactory bulb (**d, g, h**, HE), showing reactive astrocytes (arrow in **g**) and focally erythrocyte extravasation (arrow in **h**). There is prominent microglia activation (HLA-DR; **f** and arrows in **i**) and parenchymal infiltration of few CD8-positive cells (cytotoxic T lymphocytes, arrows in **j**). **k–n**: Medulla oblongata, showing prominent microglia activation (HLA-DR, **k, l**) with occasional microglial nodules (**l**). There is also evidence of albumin extravasation with its uptake in astrocytes (arrows in **m**) and perivascular infiltration of CD8-positive cells (arrows in **n**). HE: haematoxylin and eosin GFAP: glial fibrillary acidic protein, astrocytic marker; human leukocyte antigen (HLA)-DP, DQ, DR, microglia/macrophage marker. Scale bars: (**a–f**): 1 mm; (**g–i**), (**k, m, n**): 40 mM; (**j, n**) 30 mm

Another recent study provides a detailed description of the neuropathological changes related to COVID-19 in a cohort of 43 patients who died with COVID-19 in Germany [18]. Matschke and colleagues focused on the inflammatory changes and detection of SARS-CoV-2. They confirmed the occurrence of generally mild neuropathological changes, with however pronounced activation of the neuroinflammatory response, with prominent involvement of the brainstem. This is in line with previous observations, supporting the activation of the adaptive and, particularly, of the innate immune response [18]. This study does not provide evidence for CNS damage directly caused by SARS-CoV-2. Accordingly, the presence of SARS-CoV-2 did not seem to be associated with the severity of the observed neuroinflammatory changes [18].

An ongoing task for neuropathology experts is to contribute to dissect the complex pathophysiology of COVID-19 associated neurological manifestation, in particular to understand the role of a direct SARS-CoV-2 brain infection versus the sequels of an over activation of the systemic immune response, as well as the relationship between hypoxemia, diffuse cerebral micro-bleeds and coma in COVID-19 patients. In this effort it would also be important to evaluate also deceased patients with COVID-19 without significant neurological manifestations (as appropriate control cohorts). It is also essential to create a multidisciplinary team with close collaboration between neuropathology and neuroradiology. In particular postmortem MRI applied to clinically well-defined COVID-19 cases could contribute to better define the MRI signatures of neuropathological lesions in COVID-19 associated neurological and psychiatric manifestations.

References

1. Ellul MA, et al. Neurological associations of COVID-19. Lancet Neurol. 2020;19(9):767–83.
2. Rogers JP, et al. Psychiatric and neuropsychiatric presentations associated with severe coronavirus infections: a systematic review and meta-analysis with comparison to the COVID-19 pandemic. Lancet Psychiatry. 2020;7(7):611–27.
3. Al-Sarraj S, et al. Invited review: the spectrum of neuropathology in COVID-19. Neuropathol Appl Neurobiol. 2020;
4. Baig AM, et al. Evidence of the COVID-19 virus targeting the CNS: tissue distribution, host-virus interaction, and proposed neurotropic mechanisms. ACS Chem Neurosci. 2020;11(7):995–8.
5. Tassorelli C, et al. COVID-19: what if the brain had a role in causing the deaths? Eur J Neurol. 2020;27(9):E41–2.
6. Deigendesch N, et al. Correlates of critical illness-related encephalopathy predominate postmortem COVID-19 neuropathology. Acta Neuropathol. 2020;140(4):583–6.
7. Frank S. Catch me if you can: SARS-CoV-2 detection in brains of deceased patients with COVID-19. Lancet Neurol. 2020;19(11):883–4.
8. Reichard RR, et al. Neuropathology of COVID-19: a spectrum of vascular and acute disseminated encephalomyelitis (ADEM)-like pathology. Acta Neuropathol. 2020;140(1):1–6.
9. von Weyhern CH, et al. Early evidence of pronounced brain involvement in fatal COVID-19 outcomes. Lancet. 2020;395(10241):e109.
10. Solomon IH, et al. Neuropathological features of Covid-19. N Engl J Med. 2020;383(10):989–92.
11. Al-Dalahmah O, et al. Neuronophagia and microglial nodules in a SARS-CoV-2 patient with cerebellar hemorrhage. Acta Neuropathol Commun. 2020;8(1):147.
12. Kantonen J, et al. Neuropathologic features of four autopsied COVID-19 patients. Brain Pathol. 2020;30:1012.
13. Barth RF, Buja LM, Parwani AV. The spectrum of pathological findings in coronavirus disease (COVID-19) and the pathogenesis of SARS-CoV-2. Diagn Pathol. 2020;15(1):85.
14. Younger DS. Postmortem neuropathology in Covid-19. Brain Pathol. 2020:e12915.
15. Schurink B, et al. Viral presence and immunopathology in patients with lethal COVID-19: a prospective autopsy cohort study. Lancet Microbe. 2020;1:e290.
16. Bottcher C, et al. Human microglia regional heterogeneity and phenotypes determined by multiplexed single-cell mass cytometry. Nat Neurosci. 2019;22(1):78–90.
17. Alquisiras-Burgos I, et al. Neurological complications associated with the blood-brain barrier damage induced by the inflammatory response during SARS-CoV-2 infection. Mol Neurobiol. 2020:1–16.
18. Matschke J, et al. Neuropathology of patients with COVID-19 in Germany: a post-mortem case series. Lancet Neurol. 2020;19(11):919–29.

Printed in the United States
by Baker & Taylor Publisher Services